Mommy RESCUE Guide

Breastfeeding

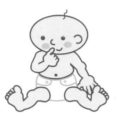

Lifesaving Techniques and Advice for Every Stage of Nursing

Suzanne Fredrogill
Certified Breastfeeding Instructor
Technical Review by Kimberly Tweedy,
R

Copyright © 2007 by F+W Publications, Inc.
All rights reserved.
Contains material adopted and abridged from
The Everything® Breastfeeding Book,
by Suzanne Fredregill with Ray Fredregill,
Copyright © 2002 by F+W Publications, Inc.

Published by Adams Media, an F + W Publications Company
57 Littlefield Street
Avon, MA 02322
www.adamsmedia.com

ISBN 10: 1-59869-332-8
ISBN 13: 978-1-59869-332-4

Printed in China.
J I H G F E D C B A

Library of Congress Cataloging-in-Publication Data
available from the publisher

Technical Illustrations by Barry Littman

*This book is available at quantity discounts for bulk purchases.
For information, please call 1-800-289-0963.*

Mommy Rescue Guide

Welcome to the lifesaving *Mommy Rescue Guide* series! Each *Mommy Rescue Guide* offers techniques and advice written by recognized parenting authorities.

These engaging, informative books give you the help you need when you need it the most! The *Mommy Rescue Guides* are quick, issue-specific, and easy to carry anywhere and everywhere.

You can read one from cover to cover or just pick out the information you need for rapid relief! Whether you're in a bind or you have some time, these books will make being a mom painless and fun!

Being a good mom has never been easier!

Contents

Introduction

WHETHER THIS IS YOUR first or fifth child, each new baby brings a set of new and different challenges. One of the most common difficulties for new mothers is breastfeeding. And that's why you picked up this book! It is perfect for a pregnant mother looking to prepare herself and her household for the breastfeeding commitment as well as the mother who is staring down at her wailing child wondering, "What should I do?" *Mommy Rescue Guide: Breastfeeding* is here to give you the lifesaving advice you need, for every stage of nursing.

The natural bonding experience of breastfeeding is one of a kind, for both Mommy and Baby, but sometimes getting the hang of it isn't so natural a process. In this book, you will find reassuring, eye-opening, and practical advice that will give you the confidence you need to be at ease with your baby at your breast.

The information in this book is current, cutting-edge, and compassionate. With expert advice on issues like getting baby to nurse, setting up a practical feeding schedule, and finding others ways to connect with your child after he or she is weaned, you can finally stop stressing and start enjoying this very special time.

Chapter 1

Why Is Breastfeeding Important?

MANY PEOPLE WONDER, "Is breastfeeding really that important?" In a word, yes! And there are many reasons why. Despite all the fantastic things humans have accomplished, we've never been able to come up with a better food than breastmilk for a baby. That's not to say we haven't tried! The formula options available can be mind-boggling. Lucky for us, the simplest choice is also the healthiest choice. No infant formula can meet your baby's needs the way your own breastmilk does. So by breastfeeding, you are doing the best thing you can for your baby.

It's Beneficial for Baby!

It's amazing to think that a mother's body produces just what her child needs to grow, build strength, and develop. As mothers, our bodies can completely nourish another being for the first few of years of life. That is a truly incredible gift! Breastmilk is the elixir of life for your baby. Each precious drop gives her exactly what she needs in just the right amounts. It's an incredible mixture that's constantly changing to meet your baby's needs. No formula can do that. While this is a natural process, it may not come naturally to everyone—but this book will help you and your baby get what you need from this one-of-a-kind experience.

Digestibility Delight

Little babies have developing digestive systems and little tummies. It's important to think about how what babies ingest will affect them. One of the greatest advantages of breastmilk is how easily your baby can digest it. This is especially important during the first year of life when your baby will be growing more rapidly than at any other time in life. Part of the reason breastmilk is so digestible is that its proteins are smaller than formula proteins. The vitamins and minerals in breastmilk are also more easily absorbed by baby's body than those found in formula or other supplements. But breastmilk goes beyond just being easy to digest.

Enzymes in breastmilk work with your baby's digestive system to help her get the most out of every feeding. As a result, breastmilk goes through your baby's system twice as fast as formula while providing her with better nourishment than any other food source.

Yes, this means that your young, breastfed baby will have more frequent bowel movements than formula-fed babies of the same age. It also means your nursing baby will want to eat more frequently than a formula-fed baby. But, your baby will spit up less and have fewer cases of indigestion. Because breastfed infants generally eat smaller meals than formula-fed babies, there's less opportunity for spitting up.

The easy digestibility of breastmilk is also important in lessening the severity of gastroesophageal reflux (GER). GER is a heartburn-like pain that happens when stomach acids back up into your baby's esophagus. There's a circular muscle where the esophagus meets the stomach that normally prevents this from occurring. However, in some babies, it takes most of their first year of life for that muscle to develop properly.

If you've ever had acid reflux, just imagine having it as a baby. Like the old Leslie Gore song says, "You would cry too if it happened to you!"

Stools: What's Normal, What's Not

As a direct result of breastmilk's digestibility, your baby's stools will be smaller, softer, and less likely to knock you out with a stench. No one is promising

Mommy Knows Best

Breastmilk is the best milk for your baby! The American Academy of Pediatrics (AAP), the World Health Organization (WHO), and the U.S. Department of Health and Human Services along with many other reputable organizations all recommend exclusive breastfeeding for at least the first six months.

that diaper changing will be like a trip to the perfume counter, but with fewer fats and proteins passing through your baby's system undigested, the smell of stools is not just reduced, it's changed.

Little Bodies

Even though your baby may look like a whole little person from the outside, until approximately four months of age, your child's immune system is underdeveloped. All sorts of viruses, fungi, bacteria, and other villains will try to invade your baby's body. Without a mature immune system, she's an easy target. But, once again, it's breastmilk to the rescue!

Many of the ingredients in your breastmilk help fight infections or promote the growing strength of your baby's own immune system. Breastmilk contains ingredients that shield the intestines, help friendly bacteria grow, keep necessary iron away from the invading cells, and cut through the invaders' cell walls.

Most amazingly, breastmilk is a living substance. Like blood, it's teeming with millions of disease-fighting cells called antibodies. These antibodies are

Mommy Must

Since you have to change your baby several times a day, you may as well become educated about what you are doing down there! Keeping track of your baby's diapers is a good way to assess your milk production. Babies typically have at least eight to ten wet diapers and four to six stools per day when they are getting enough to eat.

nature's way of immunizing your baby against every disease you have ever been exposed to. And that protection constantly improves. If you are exposed to a new germ, your body will pass on immunity to that germ to your baby through your milk. "Breastmilk immunization" can happen before you even notice the first symptoms of illness.

Adults who were breastfed as infants have lower incidences of diabetes, Crohn's disease, and coronary heart disease. Furthermore, research finds that breastmilk kills germs in babies' mouths and helps heal mothers' cracked nipples. Some moms even put it on cuts and scrapes. It's like your immune system in an easy-to-use liquid.

Growing Minds

What makes baby stronger also makes baby smarter! Your baby's brain grows at a fantastic rate in those first few months. You won't always be able to tell as she lies in your arms looking so serene, but this is her brain's busiest developmental stage. Behind that cute brow, there's a firestorm of activity. Neural pathways are forming. With

Mommy Knows Best

In June 1999, an exciting study on breastmilk and immunology was featured in "Discover" magazine under the title "Got Cancer Killers?" A protein (dubbed "HAMLET") in breastmilk causes cancer cells to commit suicide. HAMLET is reportedly deadly to "every cancer we test it against," say the researchers.

every moment, some paths are strengthened and others fade. Your baby needs the proper materials for this important work, and your breastmilk is a virtual grocery list of exactly those ingredients. Studies have found up to a 10-point IQ advantage in breastfed children.

Fats and sugars in your milk are custom tailored for brain growth. Babies need fat for brain development for at least the first two years of their lives. The fats found in your breastmilk help form the insulation on the electrical wiring of your baby's brain, and they make your baby smarter, too.

Emotional State

The connection between you and your baby during nursing is one of a kind. In fact, babies are so comfortable that they often fall asleep at the breast, full and content. Breastmilk contains ingredients that stimulate your baby's body to produce a hormone called cholecystokinin (CCK). CCK relaxes your baby and helps her sleep. It's the same hormone that makes you feel drowsy after a big meal.

The act of nursing is also comforting to your baby because it satisfies her need to suck. The skin-to-skin contact keeps her warm. Your body temperature will actually adjust itself in response to hers. Nestled in your arms, she feels safe and secure. The closeness and intimacy of the feeding experience fosters your baby's sense of trust and makes it easier for her to communicate her needs to you.

Weight Gain

We're talking about your baby's weight here, not yours! If you are looking at other babies in the nursery or doctor's office and wondering—are they the same age? Don't despair, breastfed babies generally don't gain weight as quickly in the first few days as formula-fed babies, but they soon catch up. Many breastfeeding parents are concerned that their child seems underweight according to the doctor's charts. Don't let the growth chart worry you. Those weights are based on formula-fed infants, not breastfed babies.

Formula and breastmilk generally average about the same number of calories per ounce. The difference is in the other ingredients and in the delivery system. Cow's milk, which is found in formula, is made to build body mass. The types of fats and proteins it contains encourage early weight gain. This makes sense for an animal that will gain hundreds of pounds in its first year of life. Breastmilk, on the other hand, contains a healthier balance of body and brain builders. It also changes as your baby suckles. At first, your baby gets the protein-rich foremilk. As she continues to nurse, your calorie-rich hindmilk lets down. With formula, she always gets the full-caloric version.

Facial Development

The way your baby's face develops is largely based on his sucking of your breast. In fact, babies suck differently on breasts than they do on bottles. The breast fills the mouth more completely. Breastfeeding actually works the entire mouth, while bottle-feeding exercises only the front. The sucking movements affect babies' facial development. Breastfed babies tend to have larger nasal space and better jaw alignment, which means a reduced risk of snoring, sleep apnea, and orthodontic work later in life.

Avoiding Allergies

These days it seems as if people are allergic to any and all things. But you can help your baby avoid many food allergies by breastfeeding. Allergies are blamed for problems in children and adults, ranging from the classic hay fever all the way to behavioral difficulties. Infants are especially vulnerable to food allergies because of what some doctors call the leaky gut syndrome. The cells lining a baby's intestinal walls are just not packed together densely enough at birth to stop food proteins, or allergens, from entering the body.

If you practice exclusive breastfeeding during your baby's first six months, you don't need to worry too much about food allergies. If you feed formula, however, you need to be a bit more cautious.

Mommy Knows Best

There is a yellowish fluid that comes from your breasts after birth; it's called colostrum. Many cultures have regarded colostrum as "dirty milk" and kept it from babies, but the truth is it's exactly what a newborn needs. Colostrum knocks out germs even more effectively than regular breastmilk and helps your baby get a healthy start.

Breastmilk meets your baby's needs perfectly. It contains substances that help "seal the leaks" in your baby's intestinal lining while other substances help the lining to grow. Around six months of age, your baby's leaky intestinal lining achieves "closure." As this happens, babies become less sensitive to allergens and can start trying different foods.

And It's Good for You, Too

It's time you do something for you, too! Breastfeeding has been shown time and again to have some impressive advantages for moms as well as babies. While you breastfeed, you will experience short-term benefits such as delayed menstruation, as well as reduced risks of breast cancer and osteoporosis farther down the road.

Right After Birth

If a doula or midwife assists your birth, she'll be sure your newborn breastfeeds in the first hour after delivery, even though you will be tired! Besides the fact that professional childbirth assistants nearly always advocate breastfeeding for baby, it's also an important part of your natural recovery from labor and delivery. Breastfeeding releases the hormone oxytocin, which causes your uterus to contract, thereby helping stop the flow of blood and delivering the placenta in one piece. If you choose not to breastfeed, your doctor may intervene with an injection of

Pitocin, a synthetic form of oxytocin, to aid in the delivery of your placenta.

Getting a Break

After birth and during breastfeeding, you may experience amenorrhea! Don't know what that is? Amenorrhea is big word with a little definition: no periods. Many women enjoy time off from their menses for the first six months of breastfeeding. The benefits of this little break are more than just convenience.

Lactational amenorrhea (the pausing of your menstrual cycle while breastfeeding) means reduced fertility. As long as you are exclusively breastfeeding, you're much less likely to become pregnant. With lactational amenorrhea, some women enjoy a 98 to 99 percent effective method of birth control. Best of all, it's completely natural. However, this is not an effective form of birth control for every breastfeeding woman.

The other benefit of lactational amenorrhea is the prevention of anemia. Because breastfeeding removes iron from your body at a rate of about 0.3

Mommy Must

Mother Nature has her own way of family planning: six weeks of postpartum abstinence followed by six months of breastfeeding-induced amenorrhea gives you over sixteen months between births! However, amenorrhea is different for every woman. Sometimes the shortest separation from your baby can derail the process.

milligrams per day, doctors have long considered it to be a cause of anemia in new mothers. Instead of losing large amounts of iron to your period, you can lose much smaller amounts to your baby.

Traditionally, people have viewed breastfeeding as being a "draw" on the mother's body. Today, we know that it's just not true. Breastfeeding plays an important role in helping you recover from pregnancy and childbirth.

Losing Pregnancy Pounds

How would you like to eat more and still lose weight? Wouldn't we all like that? Of course. Well luckily for you, when you breastfeed, your body will burn up the fat it stored during pregnancy to make milk. On top of that, you get to eat an additional 300 to 500 extra calories per day. You'll enjoy a good appetite and larger portions, and you'll lose pounds and inches.

Bonding

Nursing your little bundle of joy puts her close to you and gives you a chance to coo, cuddle, and take

Mindful Mommy

Breastfeeding, while always considered to be a possible cause for maternal anemia, can also provide a natural remedy. Women have a decreased need for iron after they give birth compared to when they are pregnant. And since most breastfeeding women do not menstruate for several months while nursing, their need for iron is reduced.

her in with all of your senses. We all talk about connecting with our children, and with breastfeeding the connection is real and physical. Skin-to-skin contact and suckling release stress-reducing hormones (oxytocin and prolactin) in your body that relax you and give you a calm, pleasurable feeling. Those same powerful hormones help you to literally fall in love with your newborn. Prolactin is sometimes called the "mothering hormone" because of the way it intensifies nurturing behavior.

Prolactin is also a natural tranquilizer. Within minutes of latch-on, you might begin to relax so much, you'll feel yourself getting sleepy. That's one of nature's little rewards.

Breastfeeding's Other Benefits

So breastfeeding is good for your baby, and it's good for you. And in case that isn't enough to sell you, consider the secondary effects of going au naturel. No recycling, no late-night trips to the grocery store—and, best of all, breastmilk is free!

Mindful Mommy

Keep your moods in mind. If your blues extend beyond the first two weeks following the birth of your baby, you may be suffering from postpartum depression. If you find yourself feeling lethargic, have a loss of appetite, or have a hard time functioning, contact your doctor or midwife. You're not alone and support is readily available for new mothers.

Environmentally Friendly

Breastmilk isn't made in a factory or shipped to your local supermarket. No chemicals are used to manufacture colorful labels. You don't usually need a non-biodegradable bottle or processed petrochemical nipple to use it. When you're done with a feeding, you don't have anything leftover to haul to the landfill. Maybe breastfeeding won't single-handedly save the world, but then again, every little bit helps. After all, this is the world we'll be leaving to our children.

Formula needs to be prepared and heated. Those few extra seconds can seem like an eternity when your hungry baby is crying—especially in the middle of the night. With nursing, you don't have to worry about the quality of the water or the temperature of the milk. Breastmilk is the original convenience food.

Ka-ching

Breastfeeding will save you a significant chunk of change compared with feeding infant formula:

- If you choose bottle-feeding, you can expect to spend over $1,200 annually on formula alone. If you mix that formula with store-bought

Mommy Must

Breastfeeding can give you a strong sense of accomplishment, pride, and continuity with life and the world. You don't have to be an Earth Mother to appreciate the spiritual side of childbearing or your body's ability to feed your baby. Nursing is a powerful aspect of motherhood. Trusting your body to nourish your child is a deeply satisfying experience.

water, add another $65 per year. Then you shell out more cash for the extra bottles, liners, nipples, and maybe even for dry cleaning to remove those formula-spit-up stains.

- In addition, bottle-fed babies also keep the doctors busy. By the most conservative estimates, formula-fed babies run up over $200 more in medical expenses in their first year than breastfed babies do.

- They spend more time at the doctor's office because they're sick more than their breastfed friends.

Dads Love It

Hey, new dads! As if having a happier, healthier family, a cleaner planet, and more money in your pocket wasn't enough, there's more! There are two often unspoken benefits to you that you might really appreciate: freedom from many feeding duties and an interesting new look to your already lovely partner. Breastfeeding is an experience the whole family can appreciate.

Mommy Knows Best

After nine months of pregnancy and then labor you deserve a break! One of the nicest things about breast-feeding is the convenience. The milk is always the perfect temperature, it's always clean, and you can't forget your breasts when you leave the house!

Getting to It

So now, you're convinced—breastfeeding is important. Now what? Although breastfeeding is a natural practice, learning the new skill doesn't come naturally to everyone. While some women only experience a couple of problems, others face one difficulty after another. While it may be tough at times, breastfeeding is worth the effort.

Chapter 2

Is Breastfeeding for Me?

MANY WOMEN HAVE DOUBTS about their ability to breastfeed, but you should know that the vast majority of mothers can successfully breastfeed. If you're able to give birth, you're almost certainly able to nurse your baby. There are exceptions, but they are uncommon and usually temporary. Most women who believe they were unable to breastfeed were probably just missing the two most important things every nursing mother really needs—confidence and support.

Breast Issues You May Have

Have you ever wondered if there could be something "wrong" with your breasts? If so, you have probably fallen into the trap, as thousands of women do, of believing that you are not "normal." The fact is that breast "issues" are most often a result of preconceived notions. In the past, a lack of information, education, and encouragement to breastfeed left many mothers making assumptions about why it wouldn't work for them. With the proper preparation and support, virtually all mothers can provide natural nourishment to their babies.

Breast Size Doesn't Matter

Many women think that the bigger your breasts are, the more milk you produce. But this is a myth! Breast size is mostly a matter of fat content, not milk-gland content. In fact, small-chested women may actually have an advantage over their bustier friends when nursing low birthweight or premature babies. Very small babies sometimes find it difficult to latch onto an engorged breast. In those cases, smaller breasts can be an advantage.

On the other hand, if your breasts are large and you are worried that they will just get larger, don't let that discourage you from breastfeeding. Surprisingly, large breasts don't generally get much larger with lactation. They also tend to leak less than smaller breasts.

There are advantages and disadvantages to different breast sizes, of course, but regardless of your size, stick with it, keep informed, and stay confident. You can have a successful breastfeeding experience.

Mommy Knows Best

Even if you have had pierced nipples, you can probably still breastfeed; many women throughout the years have been successful. In certain cases, piercing of the nipples sometimes scars the milk ducts and inhibits the flow of milk. If your piercings have been infected or if you have multiple nipple piercings, you may find breastfeeding difficult. All jewelry must be removed before nursing.

Nipples—They Are All Different

Like breasts, nipples come in a variety of shapes and sizes. There are:

- Nipples the size of champagne corks.
- Nipples that hide inside the breast (inverted).
- Nipples that point up, down, or sideways.

It's not unusual for a woman to have one nipple that's inverted and another that's not. No matter what type of nipples you have, breastfeeding is possible. Inverted nipples can be coaxed out and large nipples can be worked around. Other moms have done it and you can, too.

Adoptive Moms

The answer to your, and everyone's, question is yes! You can nurse your adopted baby! The process is not easy, but it can be done and has been done by many women. Your milk production can be started with the help of a breast pump and a little patience. However, initiating lactation without pregnancy requires a serious commitment.

A woman who produces milk for her own baby has the advantage of pregnancy. For nine months, her body has been preparing to feed a baby. Without those pregnancy hormones, you'll have to rely on manual stimulation as explained later (Chapter 8).

In comparison to natural mothers, adoptive moms don't usually produce enough milk to fully feed a young infant, but don't let that discourage you. Nursing your baby isn't only about nutrition. Any amount of milk you produce is a precious gift for your child and the experience of nursing will be wonderful for both of you.

Drugs and Alcohol

Without a doubt, the best practice when you're breast-feeding is to steer clear of all drugs, alcohol, and herbal products. Unfortunately, that way is blocked for some of us. Medical conditions or addictions can stand in the way of a drug-free lactation. If you smoke or drink, you'll need to make some changes during pregnancy and it is important to keep it up while nursing your child.

Will Your Medicine Effect Your Baby?

There are two questions that you should think about and consult a doctor about.

Mommy Knows Best

When you work to initiate milk production, the process is called "lactogenesis." Thanks to modern medicine, there are hormonal therapies being developed that can help a woman to lactate without pregnancy. However, these procedures may produce unpleasant side effects as well as the risk of unknown future complications. Check with your doctor.

- The first is: do the benefits to my health outweigh any risk to my baby?
- And, the second is: do I need to wean my child to protect her from this medication?

A doctor should be able to help you figure out which medications are harmless to your nursing infant and which are less safe. Fortunately, permanent weaning is rarely necessary. Although many medicines will enter your milk supply, the amounts that reach your child are usually small. As a result, breastfeeding is compatible with a wide variety of pharmaceuticals.

If you're taking a prescription drug on a doctor's order, remind your doctor that you plan to breastfeed. Some doctors routinely advise mothers to wean while medicated because they are not well informed about breastfeeding. It's often a good idea to talk to your pediatrician about prescriptions from other doctors. Your midwife or lactation consultant is also a good source of information.

While many drugs are considered safe for nursing moms, certain types are considered off-limits. Some of these drugs will affect your baby, while others can

Mommy Knows Best

If you find out that your medication is not safe to use while breastfeeding, and you decide to wean the baby temporarily, it's important to use a breast pump to maintain your milk production. You'll need to "pump and dump" as often as your baby would nurse.

decrease your milk production. Some sources consider most medications to be off-limits, while other sources consider the majority of medications to be compatible with breastfeeding.

As your baby grows, it becomes safer for you to take medications. In the meantime, take the minimum amount necessary to ensure your comfort and health. A sick mom has a hard time taking care of her child. Sometimes, you have to take care of yourself first. Consult your healthcare professional for guidance!

Okay, Maybe a Little: Alcohol

As you know, alcohol was advised against during your pregnancy, and you may have been looking forward to a glass of wine now for months. You're in luck. The rules for lactating moms are a little more lenient than they were for pregnant moms. A glass of wine with dinner or some champagne at a wedding is not completely out of the question.

However, you need to be careful.

If you have a drink, it is true that alcohol *does* find its way into your milk. The negative effects for your baby include possible long-term immunity weakness and nervous system disorders. Infants in the first months of life are especially sensitive to alcohol's effects since their livers are not yet mature enough to eliminate it easily from their bloodstream. Older babies who rely less on mom for nursing and who have more body mass are better able to tolerate small amounts of alcohol in your breastmilk.

The good news is that alcohol clears from your breastmilk at about the same rate it clears from your bloodstream. If you have a single drink immediately after nursing, your milk should be alcohol-free by the time you nurse again in two to three hours (depending on your weight).

Tradition maintains that an occasional serving of alcohol helps a mother produce more milk. Contrary to folk wisdom, however, alcohol appears to have a negative impact on successful breastfeeding. Studies have demonstrated a change in the taste and smell of breastmilk when mom drinks alcohol, and babies don't generally like it. Alcohol also reduces the levels of prolactin and oxytocin that are produced in your body when baby suckles. Prolactin aids in milk production as well as emotional bonding. Oxytocin plays a key role in your milk ejection, or letdown, response.

If you drink often, you may find your child weaning far earlier than you had planned. Your milk production, delivery, and flavor might lead to early weaning. On the other hand, an occasional drink seems relatively harmless if you allow it to clear from your bloodstream before nursing.

Stop Smoking Already

If you haven't quit smoking already, this is a great time to stop. If you're a new parent, there are some important reasons to kick the habit.

As you surely know, smoking during pregnancy leads to:

- Low birth weight
- Reduced IQ
- Heart and lung difficulties for your baby
- Increased risk of complications following birth for both mother and child

And even after delivery, smoking continues to threaten your child's health.

If you nurse your baby and smoke, nicotine will find its way into your milk. Heavy smokers (more than a pack a day) may find their babies suffer from intestinal upsets and fussiness. Heavy smokers are also nearly twice as likely as nonsmokers to have colicky babies. Like alcohol, smoking has been linked to early weaning due to lowered milk production and inhibited letdown. However, research suggests that women who smoke less than a pack a day probably

Mommy Knows Best

If you would like to quit smoking, the safest product to use is the nicotine patch. Nicotine levels in your blood are lower with the patch than they are with nicotine gum. If you choose gum, try to wait two to three hours before nursing.

won't have any dangerous amounts of nicotine in their milk.

Even if you do not smoke, make sure other adults don't smoke around your baby. Secondhand smoke is far more dangerous to babies than nicotine. Everyone needs to keep cigarette smoke far away from babies. Secondhand smoke has been linked to Sudden Infant Death Syndrome (SIDS) and respiratory infections. Just as you would insist on clean hands to hold your baby, insist on clean air for her, too.

The bottom line on smoking and breastfeeding is this: The benefits of breastfeeding generally outweigh the hazards of nicotine in your milk, but not those of secondhand smoke. If you can quit, congratulations! Your whole family wins. If you continue to smoke while nursing, you run a risk. At a minimum, try to cut down and keep the smoke away from your baby.

Taking Control, Controlled Substances

Like other drugs, controlled substances can interfere with your milk supply and letdown reflex. Marijuana, for instance, has been shown to reduce a mother's milk production by decreasing the level of prolactin she produces. It's also important to realize that any drugs you take can end up in your breastmilk, sometimes in a concentrated form. When you use, your baby uses. The damage done to a developing infant can be serious and permanent.

Street drugs like heroin and cocaine may be cut with harmful chemicals, and you can't be sure about their strength. Most importantly, recreational use of drugs impairs your ability to parent. Many drugs cause a loss of judgment and coordination. Good parenting takes a clear head.

If you have an addiction to a controlled substance, talk to your doctor about getting help.

Herbal Remedies and Your Baby

While it's always important to be careful, many herbs are safe for breastfeeding moms. You should consult your doctor about your specific regimen though because, some herbs can increase or decrease your milk supply. Others can take the place of regular, over-the-counter medications. If you choose to use herbal products, follow these guidelines:

- Check with your doctor.
- Use a brand that lists all active ingredients. The fewer ingredients, the better.
- Stick with a reputable brand.
- Check the expiration date.
- Bear in mind that tinctures contain alcohol.

While herbs may seem natural and safe, many of them are potent pharmacological substances. In fact, several of the medicines found at the pharmacy are derived from herbs. Unlike commercial pharmaceuticals, however, herbal remedies and supplements aren't tested and approved by the FDA.

Managing After Multiple Births

Two babies? Don't worry! That's why you have two breasts! You can nurse twins or even triplets without worrying about your milk supply. Your breasts are marvelous, self-regulating milk production centers. The amount of milk they make is directly related to the amount of milk removed by a baby's suckling. More suckling equals more milk.

If You've Had a Caesarean Section

Women who have delivered by C-section sometimes feel disappointed that their bodies have somehow failed them, but breastfeeding reinforces your confidence in your body's ability to nourish and nurture the new life you brought into the world. Breastfeeding is the best cure for this down-mood. Nursing your baby will help you to regain trust in your body's ability to mother while helping you to bond with your new baby. Although C-section is major surgery, and your incision can be tender, your baby can nurse without causing stress on your sutures.

Your Medical Conditions

How do your medical conditions affect your baby? It is an interesting question. You may have a chronic health concern or condition, but that does not necessarily prevent you from breastfeeding successfully. Both your obstetrician (OB) and your pediatrician can give you information on the best way to accommodate your situation while providing the best feeding option for your baby.

Diabetes and Breastfeeding

Many diabetic mothers have successfully breastfed their children. Lactating can even help you control your blood sugar during the transition from pregnancy to postpartum. You'll need to pay close attention to your diet because lactating can seriously affect your blood sugar. Keep lots of water and snacks handy when nursing to help you avoid becoming hypoglycemic. Your regular insulin injections are safe for your nursing child. Unfortunately, oral hypoglycemic medications are not safe for you to use when breastfeeding. Discuss medication options with your doctor.

Diabetes will present you with some special challenges. Diabetic moms tend to get more yeast infections and suffer from mastitis more than non-diabetics. You'll need to give extra attention to your breasts and watch out for plugged milk ducts.

You're giving your baby a wonderful gift when you nurse. Best of all, breastfeeding your baby will help her to avoid becoming diabetic, too. Studies show that breastfed babies have a lowered incidence of Type 1 diabetes as well as fewer occurrences of obesity as adults.

HIV Nursing Debate

The number of HIV-positive mothers with HIV-negative children is small, but the breastfeeding debate is huge. Some studies have found that the breastmilk of an infected woman can contain the HIV virus, but there is uncertainty about whether the virus detected is infectious. At this stage in the research, it's difficult to know what to do.

The AAP recommends that HIV-positive mothers in the United States use an alternate source of nutrition for their babies. On the other hand, many breastfeeding advocates believe that the risk of infection is so low and the benefits of breastfeeding so significant that everyone should breastfeed her baby.

A woman with HIV is more likely to be infectious if she contracts the virus during the second trimester of pregnancy or later. Babies are most susceptible to HIV during the first few months of life. If you are HIV positive and decide to nurse, take extra care of your breasts. Your baby is more at risk if you're suffering from mastitis. Cracked and bleeding nipples, along with scrapes or cuts in your baby's lips, mouth, or throat, can also result in HIV transmission.

Mommy Must

If you and your child are HIV-positive, breastfeeding will help your baby to stay healthy. Several recent studies have concluded that the immunity-enhancing qualities of breastmilk combat HIV in a baby's body.

HIV-infected women who take the drug AZT are much less likely to transmit HIV to their babies, either through birth or breastfeeding, although it does happen. If HIV turns into AIDS, breastfeeding is no longer an option. The risk of infection is simply too great.

Herpes Alert

Herpes can be deadly to newborns if a mother contracts it during the last trimester of pregnancy. If you become infected at that time, a C-section might be your only option. Herpes on a woman's breast, though, is less of a threat. With a few precautions, you can safely nurse your baby.

If you develop a herpes sore on your nipple, it's best not to let your baby nurse from that side until it's healed. Use a pump on the affected breast to maintain your milk supply. If the sore is somewhere else on your breast, cover it with a bandage or pad and continue to nurse as usual. Anytime you have an active outbreak of herpes, whether genital or oral (cold sores), you should take extra precautions. Wash your hands before handling your baby or your breasts and always keep your child away from herpes sores.

Mommy Knows Best

Tuberculosis is a scary reality for anyone, but especially a baby. The infectious disease is usually spread by adults with active TB, and children under the age of five have the greatest risk of infection. Mothers with untreated, active tuberculosis should not breastfeed their babies. Breastfeeding should not be discouraged

Cancer and Nursing

Cancer doesn't necessarily mean it's time to wean. Babies cannot catch cancer through breastmilk and many cancer treatments are compatible with breastfeeding. If you are determined, you can continue to nurse your child despite biopsies or even more involved surgeries. However, there are some treatments that can affect your ability to breastfeed. With any type of cancer, it's important that you discuss your desire to breastfeed with your doctor and follow her advice.

If your cancer treatment involves chemotherapy or the injection of radioactive compounds, you must wean your baby until those substances have left your body. Some radioactive agents remain in your body for many months. Chemotherapy drugs are among the most toxic medicines used. They will enter your breastmilk, and even a tiny amount can be harmful to your child. If you plan to resume nursing, you should pump and dump your milk until your doctor gives you the "all clear" sign. Take a look at the Medications to Avoid table at the end of this chapter.

for women being treated with first-line anti-tuberculosis drugs because the concentrations of these drugs in breastmilk are too small to produce toxicity in the nursing newborn. For the same reason, drugs in breast milk are not an effective treatment for TB disease in a nursing infant—according to the CDC, in June 2005.

If You've Had Breast Surgery

Many women today have had breast surgeries and you are not alone if you are wondering what this means for nursing abilities. The first step is to talk with your doctor about the possibility of breastfeeding your child. You might be pleasantly surprised. If it turns out that you are unable to produce enough milk for exclusive breastfeeding, don't be discouraged. Whatever amount of milk you can produce for your baby is wonderful. Every little bit contains the antibodies and nutrients that only you can provide. Remember, too, that nursing your baby isn't only about the milk. Breastfeeding is a special and loving time with your baby. If you want to nurse your child, you can purchase a supplemental feeding system. These devices allow your baby to nurse from your breast while receiving formula through tiny tubes. Another choice is to simply bottle-feed formula after each nursing session.

Breast Reduction and Milk Flow

Most women who have had breast reduction surgery can still produce some amount of milk. However, this type of surgery typically leaves women unable to produce enough milk to exclusively nurse their babies. In some reductions, the nipple is completely removed from the breast and reattached in a new location. If the nipples were completely severed, and are numb, breastfeeding is not possible. In some rare cases, severed nerves have actually grown back after breast reduction surgery, but this is very unusual. Once again, consult your doctor for some help!

Breast Augmentation

The nipple is what's important! And for this reason, in many cases, breast augmentation surgery will not usually interfere with a woman's ability to produce milk. Most surgeons make the incisions near the armpit or under the fold of the breast. With the nipple left undisturbed, nursing is generally unaffected. Some new mothers worry about implant leakage into their milk supply, but there's no need to let that bother you. The fears about leaking implants that were all over the news a few years ago have turned out to be unsupported by any valid research. Whether your implants are silicone or saline, your milk is safe for your baby.

Your Baby's Medical Conditions

You may be surprised to learn that there are a number of baby conditions that will effect your nursing plans. Although you may be in excellent health, it is possible that one of several infant conditions will present challenges for your breastfeeding plans. While most hospitals routinely screen newborns for a host of disorders, it is important that you notify your doctor if you have a family history of galactosemia, PKU, or any other hereditary conditions. A hospital lactation consultant is often available to guide you through these and other situations.

Jaundice

Jaundice is a condition that affects many newborns to some extent. Jaundiced babies appear yellow or orange because of an excess of bilirubin, a substance produced when a baby's body breaks down extra red blood cells. Jaundiced babies are often sleepy and need to be awakened to nurse. Normal newborn jaundice occurs within the first week of life and lasts no more than two weeks. Other types of jaundice may be due to medical conditions that require more advanced treatment.

If your baby is jaundiced, nursing him will help. Bilirubin leaves your child's body through his stools. Frequent nursings at the breast help your baby have frequent stools and eliminate excess bilirubin as quickly as possible.

Premature Birth and Special Nursing Needs

Preemies have special needs. They are usually very small and more susceptible to infections. They also suckle less effectively than full-term babies. To complicate breastfeeding even further, premature babies might need to be placed in the Neonatal Intensive Care Unit (NICU). With IVs and other medical procedures, nursing might not be possible.

Many parents feel helpless when their baby needs so much medical attention, but only a mother can provide her baby with the perfect food. Your breast-milk is exactly formulated for your child, whether the baby is premature or full term. There are alternative feeding methods that you can try with your preemie. Pumping will help you feel connected with your child, even when you're unable to hold her; it will also keep your milk supply up for the day she's able to nurse.

Galactosemia

Galactosemia is a rare, inherited disorder that affects about 1 in every 60,000 newborns. Babies suffering from galactosemia are unable to process galactose, one of the simple sugars formed by the digestion of the milk sugar lactose. There may be no indication of a problem when the baby first nurses. Galactosemia is only diagnosable through newborn screening. Eventually, the galactose builds up to dangerous levels.

Damage to the liver, central nervous system, eyes, and kidneys can occur. Babies with galactosemia should never be fed breastmilk or ordinary infant formulas. Your pediatrician will recommend a special diet.

Because galactosemia is a recessive genetic trait, both parents can carry the gene without any symptoms. If anyone in your family has a history of

Mommy Knows Best
Blood tests for phenylketonuria (PKU) and hypothyroidism are the only tests required by law in every state. Tests for jaundice, hypoglycemia, and sickle cell anemia are generally only performed when medically indicated. Be certain to tell hospital staff if you have a family history of any of these conditions.

galactosemia, tell your doctor immediately. Your doctor might recommend genetic counseling before pregnancy or delivery. Newborns are routinely checked in most states for galactosemia with a simple blood test. Make sure your child is tested.

Let's take a look at Kari as an example. Kari gave birth to her long-awaited daughter just before Thanksgiving. Lauren was born with meconium stain and was suctioned with a tube to clear her throat. She was slow to nurse, but suctioning, coupled with newborn jaundice, was thought to be the cause. They were released from the hospital Thanksgiving Day, after the standard newborn heel-stick.

Because Lauren had lost 10 percent of her birthweight, Kari was determined to nurse. Kari expressed her milk and finger-fed her baby. Lauren began to gain weight, but just as she was learning to feed at the breast, Kari received an urgent call from her doctor.

Eight days after birth, Lauren was identified through newborn screening to be presumptively positive for galactosemia. Ordinarily, the test results would have been back within two days. Because of the holiday weekend, it took six.

Until further testing could be completed, Lauren was put on a soy formula. For several weeks Kari expressed and froze her milk in the event that breastfeeding could continue. However, further testing confirmed that Lauren was galactosemic.

Kari has become an advocate for families affected by galactosemia. Lauren continues to thrive under her parents' informed and loving care.

PKU

Phenylketonuria (PKU) is a genetic condition found in 1 in every 16,000 newborns. Babies with PKU are unable to produce an enzyme that allows their bodies to absorb the amino acid phenylalanine. Dangerous levels of phenylalanine can build up in a PKU baby's body, causing symptoms ranging from rashes to central nervous system damage.

Babies with PKU require frequent monitoring of their amino acid levels. They need just enough phenylalanine for growth, but an excess can be toxic. Breastmilk contains lower levels of phenylalanine than regular formula but is still not safe for exclusive feeding of a PKU baby. However, a combination of breastfeeding and a special infant formula is possible for these infants. Under a dietitian's supervision, you may be able to breastfeed a little bit every day.

If you have PKU and are pregnant, you need to pay close attention to your diet. Even if your baby doesn't inherit the condition, high levels of phenylalanine in your blood can cause serious harm to your unborn child.

Mommy Knows Best

Most states require vitamin K injections, some form of eye care, and testing for galactosemia and phenylketonuria (PKU).

Some Common Medications to Avoid When Breastfeeding

Type	Comments
Antibacterials	While some are very safe, others may cause diarrhea, thrush, rash, bloody stools, and other problems. Consult your Dr. for specifics.
Antidepressants	Most common effect on infants is drowsiness, but phenelzine and tranylcypromine should not be used.
Antifungal	Ketoconazole poses some risk of liver damage.
Antihistamines	May reduce milk flow and cause drowsiness and fussiness when taken in large amounts. Especially avoid cetirizine.
Anti-inflammatory	Ibuprofen is safe, but some others are unsafe for babies under one year of age. Consult your Dr. for specifics.
Aspirin	Linked to Reye's syndrome and bleeding.
Chemotherapy	Very toxic, even in trace amounts.
Decongestants	Oral decongestants can cause fussiness. Sprays are better.
Diuretics	Most can suppress lactation.
Heart and blood pressure	Most seem safe, but acebutolol, atenolol, nadolol, sotalol, timolol may accumulate in baby's blood. Consult your Dr. for specifics.
Hormones	Hormonal contraceptives can interfere with lactation if used in the first six weeks. Consult your Dr. for specifics.
Narcotics	When given during labor, narcotics may inhibit lactation. They also cause drowsiness in nursing babies.
Pepto-Bismol	Salicylates can be toxic to nursing babies.
Tranquilizers	May make baby sleepy, but generally safe except for clozapine, which can decrease white blood cell count.

Chapter 3

How Does It Work?

NURSING IS AN AMAZING gift that mothers can offer their children. You have the incredible ability to nourish your child exclusively from your own body for the first six months of his or her life. Although you don't necessarily need to know how the process works to be a successful breastfeeding mom, you might be surprised at just how miraculous the process of lactation is.

Breast Development

Before you were even born, your breasts were developing. In fact, breast buds begin developing in female embryos just four weeks after conception. By the time of birth, basic breast development is complete. The nipples, areolas, and even some milk ducts are in place along with a small pad of fat. Everything is functional on a very small scale.

From just after birth until puberty, breast development is almost on hold. Some milk ducts and glandular tissue grow, but the process doesn't really take off until ten to fourteen years of age.

At the onset of puberty, a hormone called estrogen is secreted by the ovaries, bringing about a rush of breast development. The mammary fat pad increases in size and the milk ducts grow longer and branch out. When the menstrual cycle begins, the hormone progesterone causes the development of breast alveoli, the milk-producing cells.

By the age of twenty, the process is nearly complete. However, breasts actually continue to mature until either pregnancy or age thirty to thirty-five. Some women may wonder why, with all this growth, their breasts aren't larger. The important thing to remember is that breast development is your body's way of preparing you to nourish a baby. The size of your breasts does not affect your ability to produce milk. Breast size is actually determined by heredity and body fat, and has very little to do with your ability to nurse.

Childbirth naturally completes the cycle of breast development.

Mommy Knows Best

Some babies can leak breastmilk at birth. While it may seem strange, such leakage is normal and not uncommon. The pregnancy hormones in your body that prepare you for lactation can also cause your newborn's breasts to produce milk. The hormones typically leave the baby's body in a few days and the symptoms pass.

Anatomy of a Breast

A basic knowledge of breast anatomy is helpful in understanding milk production. Think of your lactating breasts as a kind of fruit salad. It sounds weird, but it will make sense in a minute.

The insides of your breasts are divided into sections like the inside of a grapefruit. Each of these sections is called a lobe. Every breast has fifteen to twenty-five lobes. Inside each lobe are twenty to forty smaller sections called lobules. The lobules contain the glands that produce milk. Those glands are called alveoli and they cluster together like grapes around the milk ducts. The milk ducts join together like grape stems and connect to the milk sinuses located under the areola.

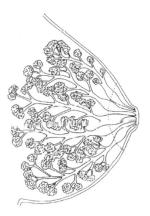

Internal Organization: The clusters of alveoli produce milk and the ducts transport it to the milk sinuses, where your breastmilk is stored until your baby's next feeding.

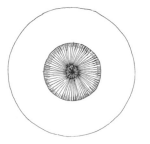

External Diagram: The breast is divided into three sections. The areola is key to successful breastfeeding.

Your Always-Changing Breasts

Your breasts will adapt themselves throughout your adolescence and adulthood in order to keep up with your life. With the onset of your first pregnancy, your breasts get their marching orders. The placenta stimulates your body to produce hormones (estrogen and progesterone) that prepare your breasts for lactation. Recent animal research indicates that the placenta itself may actually produce those hormones. Your body responds to this wake-up call in several ways.

First, your nipples and areolas darken. This helps them to stand out from the surrounding tissue and act as a visual bull's-eye for your baby.

Second, your breasts grow larger and sometimes tender. Throughout pregnancy, some women gain well over one and a half pounds in each breast as glandular tissue is being added to enable lactation. These milk-producing cells will replace a large portion of the fat cells in your breasts.

Third, your milk ducts grow. These ducts are the paths milk takes from the dairy in the alveoli to the sinuses under your areolas. Your breasts are doing road construction during pregnancy, increasing both the number of ducts and their size.

Finally, your Montgomery glands become noticeable as bumps on your areolas. These glands produce an oily substance that cleans and lubricates your nipples.

At some point in your second trimester, the prep work is done and your breasts are ready to nourish your baby. The high levels of progesterone in your body prevent lactation from occurring before birth, but you may notice a fluid leaking from your breasts. This fluid is called colostrum and it varies from thin and clear to thick and white. Colostrum is formed when the cells inside your new milk glands dissolve. Some women leak a little colostrum during pregnancy and others don't—either case is perfectly normal.

Mommy Must
Studies indicate that women who have been pregnant experience a decreased risk of breast cancer compared to women who have never been pregnant. These findings imply that your breasts are just like the rest of your body in one important way—they are healthier when used the way nature intended.

How Your Breasts Produce Milk

A breast is like a very advanced form of a bottle. But unlike a bottle, your breasts are never empty and you don't need to wait until you feel full to nurse. Milk is manufactured constantly, as long as there is demand. Milk production, or lactogenesis, normally begins with the birth of your baby. Labor and delivery start a physiological chain reaction:

Flowchart

The expulsion of your placenta causes the levels of the hormones estrogen and progesterone in your body to fall.

At the same time, nerve impulses from the uterus travel to the brain's hypothalamus gland.

The brain then signals the pituitary gland to release the hormones prolactin and oxytocin.

Extra blood is sent to your breasts so they can start manufacturing milk. It's this extra blood, along with your milk coming in, that combine to engorge your breasts, sometimes painfully.

The prolactin released by your pituitary gland causes the grapelike clusters of alveoli to produce milk.

The other hormone, oxytocin, aids in the ejection of milk from the breast.

It usually takes about seventy-two hours for your breasts to begin producing abundant milk. The process is completely under way within five days. During the first day or two of his life, your baby is nourished not with milk, but with your colostrum, the ideal first food for your infant.

Your breasts will respond to the amount of milk that is expressed. Meaning that although your milk will come in after birth whether your child nurses or not, only the constant removal of milk from the breast can maintain milk production once you begin to lactate. Your baby's suckling signals your pituitary gland to release more oxytocin and prolactin. Just like in the beginning, these hormones cause your breasts to produce milk. If your baby drinks less milk than your breast produces, the excess milk remaining in your breasts will reduce future milk production. It's a wonderfully self-regulating system.

So, if you're worried about your milk supply, the solution is simply to nurse more often. Allowing your baby to nurse whenever she wants is also the best way to increase your milk supply. If you wish to stop breastfeeding only temporarily, and hope to start up again in the future, make sure that you use

Mommy Knows Best

The more your child nurses, the more milk you produce. The less your child nurses, the less milk you produce.

a pump to express milk. If you stop, your breast will stop making milk. Supplementing breastmilk with formula short-circuits the whole process. Anything that reduces your baby's hunger or her need to suck will ultimately reduce your milk supply. That's why glucose, water, and formula are not recommended for breastfeeding babies. Your baby needs to be hungry and eager to suckle when you put her to breast.

What's in the Milk?

So what makes breastmilk so special? Why is it better than formula? Remarkably, your milk is alive. It's almost more like white blood than milk. Like blood, your milk is rich in antibodies that fight infections in your baby. Living cells from your body, called macrophages, enter your child's body through breastfeeding. These macrophages cruise through your baby's system gobbling up germs, which is especially important during the first months of life when your baby's own immune system is weak.

Your own milk also contains living enzymes that help your baby digest her meal. Formula can't do

Mommy Must

As a breastfeeding mother, you should eat milk, cheese, eggs, and meat because these foods are good sources of essential amino acids. There are twenty-two known amino acids. Eight cannot be manufactured in the body and therefore must come from dietary sources. Amino acids are clever creatures and will help your that. Neither can the cows' milk most formulas are based on. Of the hundreds of different kinds of animal milks, only human breastmilk is perfectly suited for human babies.

Your Milk Is a Baby-Friendly Food

The proteins in human milk, compared to cows' milk, are friendlier to your baby's digestive system. Most of the proteins in cows' milk are in the form of casein, which forms hard curds in your baby's stomach. Breastmilk proteins are more easily absorbed and put less strain on your baby's system. One protein, immunoglobulin A, seals your baby's intestinal track against allergens and infections. Another, lactoferrin, keeps iron away from the germs in your baby's body so they can't use it to reproduce.

The protein in our food is broken down by digestion into compounds called amino acids. Amino acids are the building blocks used to construct and maintain your body. Breastmilk contains ideal levels of taurine, an amino acid that builds and maintains the brain and eyes.

Another vital ingredient in infant nutrition is fat. Fats and cholesterol are especially important to

baby grow! They have the ability to build cells, form antibodies, carry oxygen, aid in cell reproduction and muscle operation, and perform many other tasks in the human body.

your baby's brain and nervous system development, and your breastmilk has all he needs. Human milk is your baby's only source for the important brain-builder docosahexaenoic acid (DHA). Breastmilk is also low in saturated fats and high in polyunsaturated fats. Polyunsaturated fats help build brain and nerve cells. Saturated fats only help body growth. Research suggest that adequate levels of the right dietary fats might even help reduce your child's risk of developing diseases like multiple sclerosis.

The balance of nutrients is also important. The mix of minerals and vitamins in human milk is carefully proportioned for human babies. Breastmilk provides nutrients in both a form and an amount your child's body can easily use.

Colostrum

When your baby is first born your body reacts by producing the fortifying milk that he needs, known as colostrum. It's powerful stuff! Colostrum contains more protein, minerals, salt, vitamin A, nitrogen, white blood cells, and antibodies than mature milk. It's also lower in fat and sugar. Frequent feedings of colostrum help your baby get off to a great start.

Mindful Mommy

Nature designed the breastfeeding mechanisms so well that they respond to your baby's changing dietary needs. At different times in your baby's life and even at different moments during a feeding, the composition of your milk changes.

You'll produce about two tablespoons of colostrum in the first twenty-four hours after birth. That's just the right amount for your baby's tiny tummy. In addition to the nutritional benefits, colostrum also helps clean the meconium from your newborn's intestines. Meconium causes your baby's stools to have the appearance and consistency of tar. It's a natural occurrence, but one that we're all happy to see end. The speedy elimination of meconium reduces the risk of jaundice in your newborn.

Pre-term Milk

If you give birth to a preemie, your body will know it and produce a type of milk that will help your little one grow stronger. Pre-term milk is high in fats, proteins, and sugars to help your baby grow and gain greater weight. After about a month, pre-term milk changes into mature milk. Your body's ability to formulate the right quality of milk for your baby is nothing short of amazing.

Mature Milk

A couple of days after birth, transitional milk, a mixture of colostrum and mature milk, will then lead to mature milk. Mature milk begins to come in within seventy-two hours of birth and normally replaces transitional milk completely within five days postpartum. Your mature breastmilk will exclusively provide your baby with all of her nutritional needs for the first six months of life.

Milk Ejection Reflex and Letdown

You may have heard stories about women who have milk shooting out from their breasts. You may be surprised to hear that this is not an old wives' tale—it could happen! The release of milk caused by oxytocin is called the letdown reflex or the milk ejection reflex. When your baby suckles, the stimulation to the nipple signals your body to release oxytocin, the hormone responsible for milk ejection. The oxytocin reaches your breast tissue where it causes the tiny muscles surrounding the milk-producing glands to contract. The milk is forced down the milk ducts to the sinuses beneath your areolas. When your baby nurses, she compresses the milk sinuses and the milk is pushed through the holes in your nipple

It takes a few moments after the start of nursing for letdown to occur. Fifty percent of women will know the moment it happens and 50 percent won't. You might feel a tingling in your breasts or even a "pins and needles" sensation. That feeling is followed by a sudden release of milk. Some women will experience multiple milk ejection reflexes during a single feeding. Sometimes, letdown occurs when you are away from your baby. When that happens, milk can shoot out in streams. Major tip: Nursing pads—don't leave home without them!

Once you have letdown, you'll feel thirsty, relaxed, and drowsy. You'll also feel your uterus contract. This is sometimes referred to as "afterpains."

They will decrease in intensity with time. Note: after-pains are more pronounced with each birth.

With letdown, you might notice your milk flowing faster and your baby swallowing more frequently. Even if you can't feel it, if you can see and hear your baby swallow, you'll know it's happened.

Often in the morning, when milk is most abundant, your infant may gag or cough. You can decrease the flow of milk by altering positions. Pumping for a few minutes prior to feeding will decrease the intensity of the initial flow.

Breast and Nipple Care

You have trusted your breasts all along now, knowing that they are giving your child just what she needs and when she needs it. So you shouldn't think anything different about the cleanliness of your breasts and nipples. The Montgomery glands (they may look like little pimples but don't squeeze them!) surrounding your nipples secrete an oily substance that keeps your breasts clean and moist. There is very little you

Mommy Must

If you're stressed or distracted, your letdown reflex might be delayed or inhibited. Other factors that might affect letdown include cold, pain, fatigue, caffeine, and nicotine. Fortunately, the prolactin you produce when baby suckles is a natural tranquilizer.

need to do. In fact, overzealous cleansing of your nipples can lead to problems. Soap will dry your nipple and can cause painful cracking. Soap also leaves unpleasant-tasting residue on your skin.

If you wash your hands before and after each feeding, your breasts will stay clean. After nursing, rub some breastmilk over your areola. Your milk has medicinal properties that will help keep your nipple healthy. Then, if possible, let your nipples air dry.

If you wear nursing pads, change them often. The warm, dark, and wet pad is an ideal breeding ground for germs. The best pads are washable, breathable cotton. Nursing pads with waterproof liners only hold the moisture in.

Mommy Must

Since your nipples are working to keep the nursing experience clean and healthy, do your part by using only plain water when washing your breasts. Avoid soaps and gels, even in the shower. Your nipples produce natural oils that cleanse and moisturize the areola. Soap will remove these oils and can cause problems for nursing.

Chapter 4

Am I Ready for This?

YOU MAY THINK THAT you have all you need to nurse—breasts, confidence, and a baby on the way. But it's not always that easy. Every nursing mother is bound to encounter a couple of stressful and unpleasant times. But there are some things that you can do to help you prepare for these times and get through them. Now is the time to toe up to that starting line and get set to go. You'll be glad you did.

Nipple Assessment and Prep

Know your own body before you begin; it is very important! One of the first steps toward breastfeeding success is determining your nipple type. You can do this by conducting a simple and easy nipple self-assessment. Lightly roll your nipple between your fingers, have your partner stimulate your breasts, or open the freezer door and stand in the cold air. What happens? Do your nipples stand at attention or fall back in line? Every nipple is different, even when they're on the same person. Regardless of your nipple type, you can still breastfeed. You just might need some preparation.

Inverted Nipples and How They Work

Nipples become inverted due to tight connective tissue bands under the areola. Inverted nipples appear to dent inward. (Flat nipples are caused by the same restrictive bands.) Both of these nipple types make it difficult for babies to latch on. It's still possible to breastfeed, but it might take a little extra effort. You can safely evert your nipples under the guidance of your lactation consultant. One of two methods will usually draw them out.

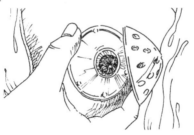

Breast shells will draw out flat or inverted nipples and may be used between feedings to protect sore nipples.

Breast shells—Breast shells are a wonderful invention for mothers who want to nurse but have inverted or flat nipples. They look like little dome-shaped cups with holes in the middle. Breast shells are worn inside your bra and fit over the nipple to put gentle pressure on the breast's connective bands and push the nipple out and through the opening. Other holes provide ventilation to keep your nipples dry.

You can wear the shells during the last trimester of your pregnancy for a couple of hours per day. Then, gradually increase to approximately ten hours at a time. Wearing the shells during labor may be helpful as well because your body has a surge of oxytocin, causing your nipples to become more pronounced. Once your baby is born, you can continue to use them. Breast shells don't hurt and no one can tell you're wearing them. They also come in handy if you have sore nipples.

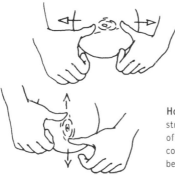

Hoffman's Technique stretches the base of the nipple and the connective tissue behind it.

Hoffman's Technique—Another method used by midwives and lactation consultants is called Hoffman's Technique. Hoffman's helps stretch the base of the nipple and gives your baby a more pliable area to latch onto. To practice this technique, place your thumbs on each side of your nipple and while gently pressing inward, pull your thumbs away from each other in a stroking motion. Now position your thumbs near the top and bottom of your nipple and repeat. You can do this several times each day during the last trimester. Ask your doctor or midwife to demonstrate this maneuver on your next OB visit.

Breast pumps—After your baby is born, you can use the suction of a breast pump to pull your nipple out just prior to putting baby to the breast, but only for as long as it takes to get the nipple erect. You need to use the pump only on the side baby has difficulty latching onto. Remember, he is feeding from the breast, not the nipple, but he must be able to extend the nipple to the back of his throat. Any breastmilk expressed by the pump can be saved for later use.

Some women with flat or inverted nipples are able to feed without any nipple preparation at all. Often, your baby will provide the best suction and the problem will take care of itself.

Nipple Preparation

In the past, some people believed that nipples should be "toughened" to prepare for nursing. But this is no longer considered best practice. Research has found that the cause of sore nipples isn't nursing friction. It's your baby's poor latch. In other words, the problem is how your baby takes the nipple into his mouth. When your baby latches onto your breast correctly, your nipples won't hurt.

The only thing you really need to do to prepare yourself for breastfeeding is become familiar with your breasts. You might not be comfortable with this at first. Women are taught to be self-conscious about their bodies from childhood, and often feel embarrassed about the size and shape of their breasts. Not only do they wear bras to support the weight of their breasts, they sometimes wear them just to keep their breasts covered.

Our society has been so successful in sexualizing breasts that we have come to believe they are purely sexual organs. Getting to know your breasts is education, not masturbation. This kind of self-exam is not unlike what women do to screen for breast cancer. All you have to do is give your breasts a mere fraction of the attention that your partner gives them and you'll learn everything you need to know. Then, you'll feel comfortable and confident that these self-regulating wonders will provide ample nourishment for your baby.

Mindful Mommy

It is possible to accidentally overstimulate your nipples during these self-assessment techniques! Nipple stimulation during pregnancy can cause uterine contractions and, potentially, premature labor. STOP if you feel any contractions. If contractions do not subside, contact your health care provider.

Social and Emotional You

So you have been going to your doctor regularly, eating and drinking all the right things, keeping active, and you feel like you are physically ready for this baby. But what about you—the emotional you? Getting physically ready for your newborn is only the beginning. It's equally important to prepare yourself emotionally for this event that will change your life forever. If someone hasn't told you this before, it's time you hear it: Once your baby arrives, life as you know it is over. For the next year or more, you will truly understand the phrase *joined at the hip*. With time, you'll wonder what life was like BC (Before Children). You will fall in love all over again and want to provide the very best life has to offer for your new baby.

Get the Supplies You Need

At some point during your last trimester, your friends and family might hold a baby shower for you. In addition to clothes, bibs, rattles, blankets, and a car seat, the items listed below would be great to have on your wish list.

A Whole New World of Bras

When you head to the mall to buy a couple of comfortable nursing bras, you'll sigh as you pass Victoria's Secret, wondering why they didn't pick up on this marketing opportunity. Then you'll head right to the granny bra section of the nearest department store. There are several styles to choose from, but your goal is to find a comfortable bra that supports your enlarged breasts and is easy to operate. Here are a few factors to take into consideration:

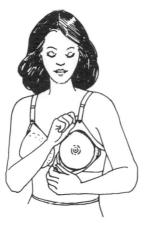

Nursing Bra:
Your bra should be supportive, comfortable, and breathable.

- Your cup size and bra (band) size will increase during pregnancy and will change when you nurse. You can expect to increase at least one size in each of these areas over the next couple of weeks.
- You'll be using the one-handed draw method for the next several months, so you'll need a bra that opens from the top to release the flap. Your new bra should also have adjustable straps, be easily breast-accessible, and refasten in a single smooth swoop. With time, you'll be able to maneuver your bra blindfolded, which

is what you'll be doing when you nurse in public.

- Comfort and support are crucial. Your bra should support not only your breasts, but part of your underarm. Your breast tissue extends beyond the obvious. Snug sports bras and other fashionable yet tight pushups will send a signal to the brain to slow milk production and can also cause plugged ducts and breast infections.

- Unless you have very large or heavy breasts, underwires are unnecessary and best avoided. They can restrict milk production and flow. If you must purchase one, select a bra that fits properly and allows for room behind and beyond the milk ducts that extend past your armpits.

- Choose a breathable cotton bra without moisture-resistant liners. Trapped moisture can breed yeast or bacterial growth. If you will be using nursing pads, it isn't necessary to have one built into your bra.

- Purchase a bra with several rows of hooks, or buy a bra extension to wear during the first two weeks. These are the straps of fabric that are lined with additional hooks that fasten to the back of your bra. They can turn a 36 band-size bra into a 40. Your breasts will change again once your routine is established, but for now you'll need a "tool" to support your expanding bustline.

When you find a bra that meets all of your criteria, buy two or three of the same kind. You'll be washing them frequently, so you'll want one available at any given time.

Pads Please

Nursing pads are a godsend for mothers with a fast milk ejection reflex. You may be standing in line at the grocery store when something triggers your letdown. Maybe it's the sound or smell of an infant. Maybe it's a picture of a baby. Your breasts may achieve letdown like squirt guns. Nursing pads are your protective barrier against public embarrassment. The most cost-effective pads are made of cotton or terry cloth and can be laundered and reused. Some are formfitting to give you extra shapeliness.

A good place to find nursing pads are department stores. You can usually find disposable pads with moisture-resistant plastic liners also. When moisture gets trapped in the liners, however, bacteria and fungi can flourish in the warm, damp darkness. Who wants a petri dish in her bra? If you're on a budget, you can use cotton hankies or cut a cloth diaper to

Mindful Mommy

Some women take pieces of a disposable diaper and cut it into sections to use as a nursing pad. But once these pieces get wet, they will release moisture beads that expand. These are difficult to remove from your breast and are easily ingested by your baby. Although the beads are not poisonous, they aren't meant for human consumption!

fit. Nursing pads just might give "stuffing your bra" a whole new meaning.

Must-Have Nursing Pillows

If you have a nursing pillow, you will love it. It can help make the experience much more comfortable for both you and your baby. You will use nursing pillows to help elevate your baby to your breast. You'll also use them to support your arms and back. Most nursing pillows will continue to be useful as your baby grows. At about five to six months, your baby can use your pillow for supported sitting.

Slings or Blankets

Slings are a must for discreet nursing in public, and they offer a convenient way to tote baby around the house. Most slings are made of a three-foot-long piece of cotton fabric that you can adjust to "wear" your baby in several positions as he grows. (Most will hold up to about thirty-five pounds.) Traditionally, slings are used in countries where women continue to work with their baby attached at the hip. In the United States, slings are a relatively new idea, but they've become the fashion choice for veteran breastfeeders.

Like baby hammocks, slings support your baby's spine and keep it aligned. Research has shown that babies carried by sling, kept close to their parents, cry less, are more calm, have stronger attachment formation, and are more in sync with Mom's movements.

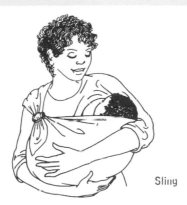

Sling

You can even wear double slings if you have twins. Think of them as baby bandoleers. The best part about slings is that you can walk around nursing your baby, and no one will know. You may opt for blankets instead, and those are just as handy. They can easily be used to shelter a nursing baby and double as warmers in a cold car seat.

Pumps Keep the Flow Going

When it comes to a breast pump, it's never too early to start researching the right one for you, and it's never too early to buy it! If you plan to return to work, or just want a reliable breast pump, make your purchase now. There are many different types and brands. You will need to choose a model that's both efficient and cost-effective. Renting is another option. Call your hospital lactation consultant, WIC office, or local breast pump depot for information. The best breast pumps are pretty pricey, but they are a good investment if you intend to use them. Some women have purchased cheap, battery-operated handheld pumps that destroy breast tissue, while others have invested in professional- or hospital-grade pumps that grew cobwebs in the closet. Again, have a good idea of what your needs are, and choose the best pump for your circumstances.

Burp Cloths

Towels and cloths are so important to have around when your little one comes! It's a time-honored truth: Babies are moist. Whether you breastfeed or bottle-feed, your baby will spit up. A couple of dozen cloth diapers are a wise, inexpensive, and necessary investment. Cloth diapers are thick, absorbent, and cost less than a new wardrobe.

Medications and Breastfeeding

Every birth is different and every mother has a different opinion about how she wants to handle it. To help ensure a positive experience, discuss labor pain management with your healthcare professional. Ask him/her what he/she recommends. During labor, you need to be free to concentrate on the task at hand and not on making last-minute decisions.

Your choices for pain relief will be either pharmacological (drugs) or nonpharmacological (nondrugs). Ask your provider to explain the risks and the benefits of the various methods she employs, as well as the effects they have on breastfeeding. A fast, relatively easy labor might require only support and encouragement. A long, difficult labor might require the use of many different options.

The most common types of pharmacological interventions include:

Morphine. Morphine is frequently used to help anxious mothers relax, or when prolonged labor is anticipated. It is administered by injection, in an IV, or in an epidural catheter. It makes Mom sleepy and crosses the placenta, making baby sleepy, too. There is often a decrease in fetal heart accelerations, and it usually slows the process of labor.

Demerol. Demerol can cause respiratory depression in both mother and baby, one of the leading causes for emergency caesarean sections. Demerol frequently causes nausea or vomiting. It also reduces available oxygen for the baby. More than any other drug used in labor, Demerol has been shown to delay initiation of breastfeeding, but that's only because someone conducted a study on Demerol and breastfeeding specifically.

Stadol and Nubain. These narcotics cause dizziness and sleepiness, after an initial buzz that sends you into space. Subsequent doses have little or no effect because your body gets used to Stadol quickly. While these medications are less likely to cause breathing problems for the baby, their relief duration is short.

Epidural anesthesia. Epidural anesthesia consists of injections of small amounts of anesthetics near the spinal nerves. This method eliminates pain in some areas of your body but allows you to remain alert throughout the birth of your baby. Unfortunately, it also weakens your contractions and slows labor. You often don't feel the urge to push and the experience of giving birth is something you might feel you have missed.

The most common types of nonpharmacological interventions are:

Pattern-paced breathing. This type of breathing is one of the relaxation techniques you learned in childbirth education class. Your mantra will start out as "hee hee hee ho" and end with "I want to go home NOW!"

Hot-and-cold therapy. The use of heated rice socks, blankets, and ice packs are natural ways to stop pain receptors from signaling the brain. They also provide competing sensations that decrease your awareness of pain.

Mommy Knows Best

Babies are affected by the labor medications even after the birth. Medication can cause your infant to have a delayed latch or uncoordinated suckling. Your baby may have a hard time getting to the breast if he's sleepy from drugs. Combining medications seems to increase this effect, especially for the first twelve hours after delivery.

Massage and acupressure. These techniques work in much the same way as hot-and-cold therapy. Acupressure stimulates a set of nerve impulses that interrupts pain signals. Massage relaxes and releases tension. Scented massage oils provide aromatherapy for the body and brain.

Changing positions. When you're medicated, you become a health risk and a hospital liability. That's why laboring women were traditionally confined to their hospital bed. Lying flat on your back throughout labor was not nature's plan. When you can walk or use a birthing ball, gravity assists you by expanding your pelvic cavity so your baby can descend more quickly and efficiently. Unrestricted movement decreases labor duration.

Water therapy. Hydrotherapy is a tool that relieves discomfort in labor. Water is relaxing in almost any form. It has proven effective in relieving high blood pressure and backache. Many women labor in the bathtub and give birth in special pools.

A large part of the decision you make about pain relief depends on your perspective and attitude about the birth process. If you are unsure about what your opinion is, consider the following question: Is childbirth a natural event or a medically managed condition?

Make a Plan, Join a Class

Many hospitals and other birthing centers encourage mothers to become involved in the birthing process as much as possible. One way to do this, is to have mothers develop a birth plan. Your doctor or midwife may ask you to do this.

Birth plans are written statements that allow you to make informed decisions about labor, delivery, and newborn procedures before your baby arrives. They are based on both current information and available options. These plans open the door for communication with your doctor. There are interactive birth plans available on several Web sites. You simply fill in the blanks, print it out, and take it to your next OB appointment.

It is important to remember that most plans are based on idealized births. Your birthing experience will almost certainly fall somewhere in the middle. You can plan for the best, but expect that there may be a revision or two, if medically necessary, and be flexible enough to allow for it.

Developing Your Plan: People, Places, and Things

When formulating your birth plan, you'll have several factors to consider, from who will be attending the birth to where you hope to have it to what labor methods you will use. Discuss your options with your partner and your healthcare professional to determine what works best for you and with your childbirth philosophies.

The People
- Who will attend your birth?
- Are partners, siblings, and extended family welcome?
- Will you use a doula?
- Will residents and students be allowed to breeze in and out during the process?
- Will your birth partner be present for all new-born care procedures?

The Places
- Will your labor take place at the hospital, birth center, or home?
- Will you labor, give birth, and recover in the same room?
- Does this room come equipped with a squat bar, birthing bed, or whirlpool?
- Will baby room with you fully, partially, or not at all?

The Things
- Will you labor naturally or use medications?
- What interventions are acceptable to you (induction, forceps, vacuum, internal fetal monitoring)?

- What labor methods are approved and supported by your provider (birthing ball, full or restricted movement, hydrotherapy)?

Remember that a birthing plan is the starting point for you and your doctor. You'll be otherwise occupied during delivery, so it's important that the other people involved know your wishes and intentions.

Your Breastfeeding Plan

It is important to be comprehensive in your birth plan. If you wish to breastfeed, you should make this clear before birth. It is important to have this in writing, but tell your healthcare professional as well as the nursery staff. If you're using a doula, she will be the first to help your baby to the breast, and she will keep hospital staff informed.

When it comes to breastfeeding, you will want to include the following in your plan:

1. Please do not offer my baby formula, glucose (sugar water), pacifiers, or artificial nipples.

Mindful Mommy

When you're exhausted and recovering from birth, your significant other is your greatest advocate! Dad can make sure your baby isn't given pacifiers, formula, or glucose, and he can stand up against hospital policies that aren't breastfeeding-friendly. At the same time, dads need to remember that nurses are busy. Treat them with respect, but make your wishes known.

2. My primary feeding preference is exclusive breastfeeding.
3. I would like the assistance of a lactation consultant or breastfeeding educator to help me establish a nursing routine before I leave the birthing facility.
4. In the event that my baby needs medical interventions, I would like to provide expressed breastmilk.

The use of pacifiers should also be identified in your birth plan. Pacifiers will satisfy your baby's sucking reflex, but you need your baby's suckle to help develop your milk supply. Pacifiers will only hinder this process. Pacifiers should not be introduced until at least six weeks after birth or until a solid nursing routine has been established.

The Use of Doulas

Many couples are now employing the services of qualified doulas to assist them with labor, birth, and postpartum care. A prenatal doula is a professional labor assistant who:

- Acts as a liaison between medical staff and the laboring couple.
- Views childbirth as a natural event and not a medically managed condition.
- Guides your birth partner in providing natural relief, support, and encouragement to you during labor.

- Helps you develop your birth plan and advocates for its use.
- Provides comfort measures.
- Records all aspects of your birth story.

Both moms and dads report more favorable birth experiences with the use of a qualified labor assistant. Dads often find the experience much more positive and pleasurable and far less stress inducing when another person is present to share the task of providing comfort and support.

Both prenatal and postpartum doulas are available to help you establish a breastfeeding routine. Your prenatal doula won't leave your side until your baby is placed at your breast and has latched on properly. Your postpartum doula will assist with newborn care, breastfeeding, emotional support, and, sometimes, light household assistance. They provide home-based services because home is the environment where you will raise your baby.

Most doulas charge between $200 and $800 per delivery and accept payment on a sliding fee scale or through a payment plan. Currently, Doulas of North America (DONA) is working on insurance

Mommy Knows Best

Studies on the use of doulas have found a 50 percent reduction in Caesarean rates, 25 percent decrease in labor duration, 30 percent decrease in the need for labor medications, as well as fewer birth complications, lower rates of postpartum depression, and greater reported satisfaction with the childbirth experience.

reimbursement for families who use this service. You can find a certified doula by contacting DONA, your childbirth educator, or your doctor or midwife.

Breastfeeding 101

There are many classes that offer tips and solutions for breastfeeding women. Breastfeeding classes are offered at your local hospital, through private maternal health organizations, or through your local WIC office. WIC not only offers classes for low- and middle-income families, but it can also refer you to local resources that support breastfeeding.

Most hospitals offer breastfeeding classes free of charge once or twice per week. Some classes are offered for pregnant couples who want more information about the techniques involved in nursing infants, while other classes focus on common concerns you have with your newborn. You might attend both. Postpartum breastfeeding classes offer one-on-one support with lactation consultants who answer questions and demonstrate new techniques.

Choose a Pediatrician

If you know for sure that you want to breastfeed, do your research and find a pediatrician who supports the practice. Almost all do, but some are too quick to offer formula or weaning as solutions when other options are available. The AAP has published its philosophy about the benefits of breastfeeding and it encourages mothers to nurse for six months exclusively and for as long as they want to after that.

It's important to find a pediatrician who has a wide knowledge base about breast anatomy, as well as personal experience with breastfeeding in general. Ask your provider why he supports breastfeeding, who he makes referrals to for potential problems, when he recommends weaning, and how many breastfeeding families are involved with his practice. Your provider will develop a health history with your child over the next several years. You can afford to be picky about who you will partner with.

Chapter 5

How Do I Do It?

THE FIRST FACE-TO-FACE MEETING with your baby is a moment that you will never forget. Barring any complications, immediately after birth, your doctor or midwife will lay your newborn on your tummy and you'll greet each other for the very first time. Your baby will be alert and the sound of your voice will captivate her. She will turn her head to listen to her mommy and daddy, and your voices will calm her cries within seconds. She might even try to vocalize in response to your soothing coos.

At First, at the Hospital, at Home

Your breastfeeding regimen will begin immediately after birth. If breastfeeding is in your birth plan, your nurse or midwife will place your baby at your breast to help involute your uterus and expel your placenta (or afterbirth). Nipple stimulation from your baby's suckling will cause your uterus to contract, which will gently squeeze the placenta to separate it from the uterine wall. It takes usually two to five contractions to deliver the placenta. Oxytocin is produced naturally when your baby nurses; it helps the uterus to contract, which controls blood loss and the risk of hemorrhage.

While your care provider is busy delivering the placenta, clamping and cutting the umbilical cord, repairing any tears to the perineum, and completing documentation, you and your baby will be exploring each other through rich sensory contact. You'll be counting her fingers and toes, and she'll be committing your scent to memory. Studies have shown that babies can identify their mothers from just the smell of their milk. Your baby is also satisfying her sucking reflex. This is the beginning of a beautiful relationship that will last a lifetime.

At the Hospital

After your baby is born, it's time to meet with a lactation consultant. A lactation consultant is a professional in the art of breastfeeding. Lactation consultants take international board exams to become licensed to practice, just as lawyers take the bar exam to practice law. They're recognized as top-level professionals in their field.

Mommy Knows Best

You may wonder, how does my baby know what to do? Well, newborns are hardwired for breastfeeding. They can zero in on the darkened bull's-eye of the areola. Babies nuzzle the nipple aggressively to make it erect for latching on. They also have the ability to "crawl" to the breast within the first hour after birth and to memorize the smell of your breastmilk.

Most hospitals have a lactation consultant on staff, but in smaller or rural facilities, postpartum care nurses or certified breastfeeding educators will assist you if a lactation consultant is unavailable. These talented and caring people are there to instruct you in every aspect of breastfeeding, from positioning to latch to assessment. They'll show you how to nurse your baby and will provide support because they want you to succeed! If you happen to have a video camera handy, tape their demonstrations. They'll be invaluable when you go home and are on your own. Here are some key points:

Don't Be Afraid to Ask a Question

- No question is too silly, stupid, or small. If the answer is vague or you just don't understand, ask your lactation consultant to slow down and speak in real-world terms. Don't hesitate to seek clarification. Have Dad, your labor coach, or another support person take notes for you or take this book with you and jot notes in the margins.

Watch and Learn

- Observe and pay close attention as your lactation consultant or nurse demonstrates positions and steps involved in putting your baby to your breast. You'll have the opportunity to practice nursing several times before you leave the hospital.

At Home, Alone?

When you first arrive home with your new baby, you might feel a little nervous or awkward about breastfeeding on your own. "Test anxiety" is perfectly normal when you're doing it for the first time on your own.

First and foremost, relax! Feel confident in your ability to do this! Keep this book close by for reference and feel free to contact your postpartum care nurse or lactation consultant for a final run-through. The first couple of weeks take practice, but by the time you go in for your postpartum checkup, you'll have nursing down to an art.

When to Feed

In the first couple of weeks of your baby's life, you will receive both advice and a lot of questions about how you are nursing. Whether the advice is wanted or not, realize that every mother-baby relationship varies. When it comes to postpartum care nurses or lactation consultants, you will be expected to explain your nursing routine. You'll be asked if you are feeding

Mommy Must

If there's a time to be a bit selfish, this is it! If you are unclear about anything, ask again. Don't be intimidated by a busy hospital or a hurrying nurse. This is your time. What you learn now can determine your immediate breastfeeding success.

on schedule or on demand. *On demand* is a term used to describe your baby's biological cycle. *On schedule* usually means by the clock. In the first few days after birth, you will be doing both.

Frequency

It will be interesting to see how often your baby expresses a need to eat. If you decide to feed on demand, how often you feed will be determined by your baby. If she is allowed to follow her own body rhythms throughout her life, she is less likely to be an overweight adult. Feeding on demand will also establish a strong milk supply. Babies know when they are hungry. They will demonstrate hunger cues when they are ready to eat. Put simply, babies eat when they are hungry and they stop when they are full. The only clock your baby cares about is her own body clock.

Keep in mind, babies in their first week of life are very sleepy, particularly if labor medications were used during the birth process. If your baby isn't waking on her own every two to three hours during the first week, you'll need to wake her to breastfeed. If you need to do this, you are feeding on schedule or "by the clock."

Mindful Mommy

Watch your baby closely during the first week of her life. If, after a week, your baby is still very sleepy, take her to your doctor or midwife for a jaundice assessment. If she has yellow skin, yellow in the whites of her eyes, brick-red or dark urine, pale stools, or feeds poorly, she might need bilirubin lights, a form of phototherapy.

After the first week of life, your baby will be more wakeful and will begin to tune into her own body rhythms. Until then, you will have to rouse her to reinforce the feeding pattern.

Schedule

During the early days, you'll realize that there is no schedule. Your baby has her own internal gas gauge. She has been inside your body for nine months now, and she doesn't know when it's day and night, or when it's meal time. Instead, her body will tell her when she's hungry and she'll show you by demonstrating hunger cues. Your baby is ready to eat when she exhibits these behaviors:

- Brings her clenched fist to her mouth
- Begins sucking on her fist or fingers
- Roots by turning her head to find your nipple
- Displays increased activity or movement
- Vocalizes and begins to make noise

Crying is a late hunger cue. If you wait until babies cry, you've waited too long. Identifying early hunger cues is an important part of learning to "read" your baby's behavior. Knowledge is power. Anticipate that she will be hungry when she wakes up, or when she displays these cues.

How Long to Feed

How long is too long? Should I cut my baby off? These are all good questions! The common practice is to offer one breast first, and when baby is finished, offer the second. Women were once advised to let their babies nurse for just ten minutes at each breast. Recent research suggests that the ten-minute rule no longer applies. The composition of breastmilk changes during a single feeding session and your baby needs both the foremilk and the hindmilk you produce. The foremilk comes quickly and is higher in volume and protein and lower in fat. The hindmilk is higher in fat and calories, but there's less of it. It's like having steak and ice cream, dinner and dessert. Babies need both.

Alternate the starting lineup at each feeding Your baby might prefer one breast to the other, and that's normal. It might have to do with the position you hold her, the flow of milk, or any number of factors. You might prefer one breast to the other for the same reasons. However, it is essential to alternate your breasts to ensure a good milk supply.

Feed for as long as your baby is interested, fifteen to thirty minutes on average. If your baby is a marathon nurser on one breast, it could indicate that she is not latched on properly or that there's a problem with

Mindful Mommy

Instead of the old ten-minute rule, today, most experts will tell you to feed your infant for fifteen minutes on each breast. Though, the key is to watch your baby and not the clock! It's more important for your baby to remove your milk than it is to follow a predetermined time limit.

your milk supply. However, babies approach nursing differently. It's a lot like eating ice cream . . . some of us lick and savor, while others bite and swallow. It rarely takes more than a maximum of twenty minutes per breast to "empty" it. Some babies will continue to nurse for comfort.

Breastmilk is very digestible, so breastfed babies eat more often than formula-fed babies. In the first weeks, your baby will eat smaller amounts, but frequently. Later on, your baby will eat more and will reduce the number of feedings. Growth spurts happen around three weeks, six weeks, three months, and six months, and usually last about seven to ten days. During this time, you might notice that your baby eats more, and more frequently. Frequent feedings not only satisfy your baby, but they tell your body to make more milk in preparation for your baby's growing demands.

When Your Baby Is at Your Breast

Finally, you are doing it! And although it may be awkward or you may be anxious at first, before you know it both you and your baby will be old pros. Until you've mastered your technique, however, follow these simple steps for successful breastfeeding. With practice and patience, you'll be nursing like a pro in no time!

Getting Ready

Before you sit down to nurse with your baby, wash your hands! It's like any other mealtime. As discussed, the Montgomery glands will keep your nipples clean, but it's essential to practice good hygiene when handling both your breasts and your newborn.

Also, don't forget your water! There's something about nursing that makes women thirsty, so have a beverage available. Water is the best choice, but juice or decaffeinated teas are healthy, too. Avoid caffeine, as it can reduce your milk supply and cause tummy upset for your baby.

Next, find a comfortable place that will become your nursing nest: a couch, a rocker, or your bed. Use pillows to support your elbows, arms, and back. Use a footrest, a telephone book, or last week's laundry to support your feet. Rocking chairs with footrests are perfect, but feel free to improvise with what you have available. It's important that you're comfortable. You may be there for a while.

Your Co-Star

This is it—time for you two. It can feel like you and your baby are the only two people in the world. And a feeling like this probably won't last! So bring your baby close to you, chest to breast, using the position that works best for both of you. Your baby's body will face you. Use pillows to bring her up to the level of your breast. Nursing pillows, bed pillows, rolled blankets, baby slings, or couch cushions will offer your baby support and the height she needs.

It's important when you are chest to breast with your baby that her ear, shoulder, and hip form a straight line. Turn your head and try to swallow. It's not easy and it's uncomfortable! That's why it's important to have your baby's body aligned (ear, shoulder, hip).

Support your breast with a C hold, like the way you hold a hamburger, only upside down. When we eat, we use our hands to shape and contour the sandwich. The same principles apply here. Support your breast with your thumb on top, positioned behind the areola, and the weight of your breast in your hand. After a while, you might not need to continue this hold throughout the entire feeding, but if you have large or heavy breasts, they'll benefit from the support. If your hand seems awkward, place a rolled up towel under your breast for support.

The All-Important Latch

Once your baby latches on, she will be able to get the proper nutrients that she needs. But if the latch is not a good one, she will struggle to get any milk at all! Encourage your baby to open her mouth as wide as possible, as if she were yawning. You might tickle her cheek or bottom lip to stimulate her rooting reflex, if

Mommy Must

The motion of pulling your baby toward you is very important. Instead of leaning down to your baby, bring your baby to your breast. With one hand cradling her head, your forearm supporting her back and hips, and the other hand holding your breast, pull your baby to you.

needed. In one sweeping motion, pull baby toward you to position her at your breast. Center your nipple over your baby's tongue, aim your nipple toward the roof of her mouth, and bring her chin to your breast.

Latching on correctly is the most critical key to breastfeeding success. This part takes some practice. Your baby should take the entire nipple and most of the areola into her mouth. If you have large areolas, make sure she's getting about one inch of it into her mouth. More areola should be visible at the top of your breast than at the bottom. Latching on is not symmetrical. Note where her lower lip makes contact. It's the lower jaw that actually extracts the milk as she compresses the milk sinuses. Your nipple should be centered over her tongue. If it just doesn't feel right or it hurts, pull baby's lower lip back enough to see if her tongue is properly positioned over her lower gum line. If you can't see it, or if you hear a clicking noise when she nurses, she might be sucking her tongue in addition to your breast. Break the latch and reposition her on the breast.

Your baby will take your nipple to the back of her throat. As she works her bottom jaw to compress the milk sinuses, milk trickles down the back of her throat. It's similar to the way you would suck your thumb.

Breaking the Latch

Break the latch by inserting your finger into your baby's mouth at the inside cheek to release suction. Hook the nipple and draw it out as you pull your breast away. Baby might try to relatch, but if your hooked finger is covering your nipple, she can't.

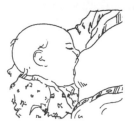

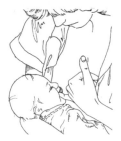

A Proper Latch: Your baby's mouth will cover most of your areola.

Breaking the Latch: Insert the tip of your finger between your baby's lips and your breast to break the suction.

If you allow your baby to slide off the nipple while she's still creating suction, you'll have sore or cracked nipples. Breaking the latch will be a smooth process once you have tried it a couple of times.

Latch Evaluation

- Does your baby have the entire nipple and at least one inch of the areola in her mouth?
- After your milk lets down, can you hear your baby swallow?
- Does baby follow a "suck, suck, suck, swallow" pattern?
- Do you hear a clicking sound that indicates improper latch?
- Can you see noticeable movement in her jaw all the way to her ear (ear wiggling)?
- Is the area at her temple moving?
- Are her lips everted around the nipple?

If you are in pain, something is wrong! Breast-feeding should not be painful. If your baby is positioned on your areola correctly, you should not feel anything more than a slight tug. Pain is often the result of nipple feeding, and continued nipple feeding will lead to cracked or sore nipples and even greater discomfort.

Suck, Suck, Suck, Swallow

Babies follow a rhythm, like a beat in a song. At first they suck steadily and somewhat aggressively to stimulate your milk ejection reflex. As the jaw moves up and down against the breast sinuses to extract milk, you'll begin to notice a pattern to your baby's nursing—suck, suck, suck, pause. She might suck from four to ten times, pause for about five or ten seconds, then continue this pattern for about three to five minutes. This pattern stimulates the letdown of your hindmilk. Once this happens, you will be able to hear her swallow.

- Her rhythm changes to suck, suck, suck, swallow, pause, suck, suck, suck, swallow, pause.

Once breastfeeding is established, letdown happens more quickly. The flow of a fast milk ejection reflex can sometimes be more than your baby can handle. You might notice milk dripping from her mouth or she might cough and need to catch her breath. Read your infant's cues. If she's sputtering, break the latch and take her off the breast just long enough for her to swallow, then begin again. After a few minutes you'll notice that her suck will begin to slow and she'll have longer pauses between sucks.

As babies tire and begin to nod off, there will be several very long pauses. But the minute you try to take your baby off the breast or stimulate her cheek, she'll almost always start to suck again. Often, by this time, baby has slid off the areola and is nipple feeding, not breastfeeding. Break the latch and start again.

Contractions: Oh No, Labor Again?

Early on, you will feel uterine contractions when your baby begins to nurse and this is normal! These contractions are called after-pains. You might feel a gush of blood on your sanitary pad at the same time. With nipple stimulation, your uterus regains its tone and dispels excess blood. These same contractions also shrink your uterus to its pre-pregnant pear size.

If this is your second or third baby, your contractions might feel stronger than before. Take a breath or practice the breathing patterns you used in childbirth education classes. After a few weeks, these contractions will cease.

Ending a Feeding

When your baby is done with the first breast, burp her, change her diaper if necessary, then offer her the second breast. However, she might fall asleep without finishing the second breast. But unlike a bottle, your breasts are never empty. If your baby falls asleep, remember to start on the unfinished side the next time your baby nurses.

Breastfeeding Positions

You and your baby should experiment in the first couple of days to find which position suits you the best. Don't be discouraged if it takes a little time, both of you will find a technique that works. You'll also discover your preference for positions after some practice. It is important that you feel comfortable with at least one of the positions listed below. Here are a few different options for you to try.

Cradle Position
The cradle position is the most commonly used breastfeeding position during the first few weeks of life. Because we tend to be cautious about holding our newborns, we tend to choose positions that allow us more control. In the cradle position, as in all breastfeeding positions, the baby's ear, shoulder, and hip will form a line and baby will be chest to breast with you.

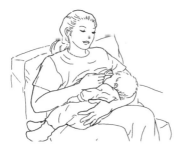

Cradle Position

Cross-Cradle Position

This is another excellent method and the one used most frequently while learning the art of breastfeeding. The cross-cradle gives you maximum control in holding your baby and bringing her to the breast. If nursing on the right side, gently place your left hand behind your baby's ears with your thumb and index finger behind each ear. Your baby's neck rests in the web between the thumb, index finger, and palm of your hand. The palm of your hand is positioned between her shoulder blades. Your right hand supports your breast in the C position.

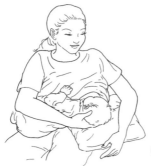

Cross-Cradle Position

Football Hold

This is an excellent position for a mother who has had a Caesarean birth, has large breasts, or has a very large baby or a premature baby. Most newborns are comfortable in this position, too. To use the football hold, place baby on her side at your side. You will support your baby's head in your hand and her back along your arm as you did in the cross-cradle hold, but this time the baby is beside you and her legs are tucked under your arm. Continue to support your breast with a C hold using the opposite hand.

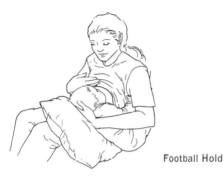

Football Hold

Side-Lying Position

Many moms use the side-lying position to nurse their babies at night or if they are on bedrest for medical reasons. In this position, you can bring baby to bed with you and nurse while lying down. Both you and your baby lie on your sides facing each other, chest to breast. Baby is cradled in your arm with her head in the crook of your elbow. Her back is supported by your forearm, on the same side you're nursing her on. Baby's hip, shoulder, and ear form a line. Use pillows to support your head, back, and legs during this feeding. If you are anxious about trying this position at night, practice during the day until you feel more comfortable. Roll up a towel or blanket to place behind your baby to support her back.

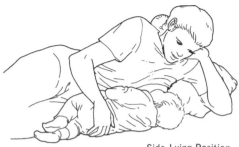
Side-Lying Position

Using a variety of positions helps to work the breast from all angles and empties the breast more efficiently, reducing the risk of plugged ducts. With time, you and your baby will find a feeding pattern that works best for you. Perhaps you're right-handed and have found the cross-cradle position on the left breast most comfortable and the football hold on the right breast the best position. You don't need to be an expert with every one of these breastfeeding positions. Feel free to mix and match whichever position works for you.

Mommy Knows Best

You can practice positioning with a doll before you have your baby to get the hang of it. Even though you will take cues from your baby when she arrives, it can't hurt to see what makes you comfortable. Don't wait until the last minute—breastfeeding is a learned art, and practice makes perfect.

Fine-Tuning Techniques

If your baby is eating and you are happy, then congratulations! Now that you have the basics down, there are some fine-tuning techniques to help make the next couple of months (or years, depending on how long you choose to breastfeed) more relaxing. Think about the following things:

Burping cloths—Keep your supply of burping cloths close by. You might use several at each feeding in the first few weeks, so have at least a dozen or so within easy reach of your chair or bed.

Chair—Whether it's a stuffed recliner, a decorative glider, or a wooden rocker, your chair should be comfortable. You'll need support for your back and arms as well as your legs.

Climate—Your home should be kept at a temperature that's comfortable for everyone. Your nursing nest should be strategically placed away from drafts in the winter and hot or stuffy spots in the summer.

Drink—Take one with you and keep it within easy reach. It's inevitable that you'll become thirsty when your baby starts to nurse.

Lighting—Try to pick a location that allows you to control the lighting. You'll want to keep the room dimly lit at night and at nap times. Bright lights don't seem to bother nursing babies, but they might make it more difficult for you to relax.

Magazine—Reading a magazine or a book while your baby nurses is a pleasant way to pass the time.

Music/TV—Listening to music or watching your favorite shows can help you relax. If you have a remote to work the stereo or TV, all the better.

Pillows—You'll need pillows for support as well as to raise your lap.

Table—You'll need a table to hold your drink, remote control, book, and perhaps a breast pump.

Like sitting down to do anything, getting settled to breastfeed will require a bit of planning and a bit of compromise. You'll forget the phone, or the remote control, or the nursing pillow. You'll know soon enough which accessories you can live without—and which are critical to success.

Establishing a Routine

In the first couple of weeks, you might think that a baby routine simply sounds oxymoronic! And as days melt into nights and you're walking in a twilight slumber, you'll wish your newborn knew what routine meant. But with the passing weeks, things will change and your baby will develop a fairly predictable schedule for eating, sleeping, playing, and eliminating. You'll become more in tune with your infant's cues and able to anticipate what will follow next.

There is value in routines. They give adults some sense of control, and as children get older, routines promote good habits and give kids a feeling of security and structure.

The Early Days

It is normal for a baby to be sleepy in her first two weeks of life. But it is necessary that she eats! So don't be surprised if you have to wake your baby every two to three hours to feed, particularly in the first two weeks. You'll offer your baby your breast eight to twelve times in every twenty-four hour period. Demand feeding won't begin until after your sleepy baby has had time to regulate her internal body clock, about two to three weeks after birth. At that time, you'll breastfeed as often as your baby wants. It might be anywhere between one and four hours, or it might be a series of evening cluster feeds. Your baby will let you know when she's hungry. However, during those early sleepy days, you'll be waking her to ensure that she has plenty of opportunities to eat, drink, and be merry.

Around three weeks of age, some babies want to nurse every hour, particularly if they are entering a growth spurt. These frequent nursings are called cluster or bunch feeds. Babies seem to space their feedings closer together at certain times of the day or night, then wait long periods between nursing sessions. It seems that just as you're ready to take

Mommy Knows Best

Many mothers worry if their babies are getting enough nutrients from just their breastmilk. They are! In fact, supplemental feedings of formula are unnecessary. While cluster feedings can be unnerving, they are a natural way for your baby to stimulate increased milk production, and for your breasts to meet the demands of your growing infant.

your baby from the breast, she begins to root again. Cluster feeds are usually followed by longer periods of uninterrupted deep sleep, a sign that your baby is going through a growth spurt. Cluster feedings can cause a new mother to wonder if she's producing enough milk for her hungry baby. They can also try a mom's patience, but the phase is usually temporary (until the next time).

This is the way you will be developing your newborn "routine" for the next couple of weeks:

Routine	
You will watch your baby.	Your baby will give hunger cues.
You will position your baby, breast to chest.	Your baby takes position to nurse.
You prepare to latch baby to your breast.	Your baby latches on.
You drink to thirst.	Your baby nurses to satiety.
You feel sleepy.	Your baby feels sleepy, too!

When your baby begins to doze or flutter-suck after feeding for some time, burp her and offer her the second breast. Your baby will probably have a bowel movement once or twice during the nursing session. The diaper change can correspond with the breast switch. It might take up to three weeks before you learn to read your infant's cues well, but you will. Soon, you'll be a pro at interpreting even her most subtle of cues, as only a parent can.

When Your Baby Sleeps

In their first two weeks of life, babies eat and sleep, eat and sleep, eat and sleep. In their first week, they sleep an average of twelve to twenty hours per day.

Sleep Chart

Week	Day	Night	Total
First Week	8–10	8–10	16–20
One Month	7–10	7–8	14–18
Three Months	6–8	6–8	12–16
Six Months	4–6	6–8	10–14
Nine Months	3–5	8–10	11–15
Twelve Months	2–4	8–10	10–14

This sleep schedule indicates hours of sleep in a twenty-four-hour period, not consecutive hours of sleep! If you manage to get four uninterrupted hours of sleep, count yourself lucky. Baby-care shifts work well during the early weeks, so both you and your partner have an opportunity to sleep undisturbed for a short period of time. Night sleep patterns do not mean after midnight, either. "Night" is anytime after the sun goes down. Sleep time will increase at night as your baby begins to eliminate naps.

Mommy Must

Even though your baby is small, it's important to change her positions and environment often throughout the day. Rocking, singing, talking, taking walks, massaging, playing on the floor, and being carried by sling all help to offer opportunities for your baby to explore! Intelligence is built like a pyramid. The broader the base, the higher the peak.

Waking Your Sleepy Baby

As mentioned earlier, babies spend their first two weeks in a sleepy state, and therefore they must be awakened every two to three hours for feeding. Frequent feedings mean a more abundant milk supply for you and healthy weight gain for your baby.

It may seem counterintuitive to wake your baby, but here are some tricks to get her up and eating!

- Change her diaper or gently wipe her face or back with a cool washcloth.
- Gently stroke her mouth, cheeks, and lips.
- Hold her skin-to-skin with you or Dad.
- Hold her upright, under her arms, and, while supporting her neck and head, gently bounce her, sing to her, or offer her your clean finger to stimulate her sucking response.
- Lay her on her back and stimulate her skin with massage.
- Rub the palms of her hands and the soles of her feet.
- Try scalp massage by drawing small circles on her head with your fingers.

If it's the middle of the night, and you want to go back to sleep after nursing her, you can nurse her while she is still sleepy. Instead of rousing her completely to a wide-awake state, keep the lights low and block out external noises that might startle her. She needs to be alert enough to nurse but not so much that she has a hard time falling back to sleep.

Middle-of-the-Night Feedings

Perhaps the biggest adjustment new parents must make is their sleep schedule. Before your baby was born, you slept when you were tired and stayed in bed as long as you wanted. Now, the amount of sleep you get will depend on your baby.

Your newborn doesn't have a set schedule, and even after he does, you'll be up several times in the night to feed him. The quality of your sleep will change. You'll sleep more lightly, almost with one eye open and one ear to the baby monitor. If you are co-bedding, every little stir will rouse you.

If you're expressing milk, trade nights with Dad or take shifts. You can work 10:00 P.M. to 2:00 A.M., and he gets 2:00 A.M. to 6:00 A.M.

Most babies wake two to three times to be fed throughout the night. Some sleep in four-hour stretches. Keep external stimulation to a minimum, unless you're trying to wake a sleepy baby for a feeding.

Around six or seven months of age, or when solids are introduced, babies will often begin to sleep through the night. If they're offered a varied diet during the day, they might not need to feed at night as

Mindful Mommy

A safe sleeping environment is important! Make sure to do the following things: always place her on her back on a firm mattress. Don't use overstuffed blankets or comforters. Remove pillows and toys from your baby's crib. Keep the room temperature comfortable, neither hot nor cold. Dress baby for sleeping the same as you would dress yourself.

frequently as before. There's no hard and fast rule, though. Your baby will let you know when he needs to nurse.

The Family Bed

Co-bedding has been a cultural practice for all but a few Western societies since the beginning of time. Japanese, Chinese, Indian, and other cultures shared beds with newborns as a way to give babies shelter and security. Even in the United States in times past, parents shared their beds with infants and toddlers.

Popular Opinion

Co-bedding isn't for everyone. Some people, especially breastfeeding moms swear by it, but among others the practice has received mixed reviews. Breastfeeding mothers describe feeling more in sync with their co-bedding infants. They share the same sleep cycles, and mothers often report feeling more rested as a result. It is easier for a co-bedding baby to breastfeed and return to sleep, without completely entering an alert state. Mothers simply gather their infants in their arms and side-lie as their

Mommy Must

It is far more pleasant to have your body wake you up than to hear the clamoring sound of an alarm clock in the middle of the night. So, drink a full glass of water at bedtime. When you get up to go to the bathroom, pick up your baby for his night feeding. If you break into his sleep rhythm before he has a chance to fully wake up, you'll be able to get him back to sleep more easily.

babies nurse at the breast. Co-bedding moms often approach nighttime feedings with a relaxed attitude, mind, and body which in turn helps their milk ejection reflex.

SIDS and Co-bedding

The family bed might even help reduce your baby's risk of sudden infant death syndrome (SIDS). Co-bedding studies by Dr. James McKenna indicate that infants co-bedding with their parents spend greater time in active or light sleep than infants who sleep alone. SIDS most often occurs when infants are in a state of deep sleep.

Don't place babies on waterbeds, beanbag chairs, or padded mattresses. Remove all pillows from around your infant, as well as blankets and comforters. Bed sharing, or co-bedding, by itself neither causes nor prevents SIDS.

Make Sure It's a Safe Co-Bed

In the past, doctors have stated that parents instinctively know not to roll over on their babies. Apparently, the same subconscious awareness that keeps you from rolling off the bed keeps you from

Mommy Must
If you co-bed with your baby, make sure your sleeping environment is as safe as her crib to prevent the risk of SIDS.

rolling onto your baby. Still, there are precautions you should take.

Make sure that your bed is not overcrowded. Toddlers should not sleep with infants. They thrash in their sleep, often turning sideways in bed without any conscious awareness of it. Likewise, dads should not sleep next to the baby. Men tend to sleep more soundly and may not be aware if they have thrown an arm over their infant, trapping them against the mattress.

Also, parents who use drugs or alcohol should not co-bed with their infants. The risk of suffocation is far greater when a parent is under the influence. Drug and alcohol use interfere with your natural ability to sleep lightly with your baby.

Sudden Infant Death Syndrome (SIDS)

Sudden infant death syndrome is a tragic occurrence. SIDS is the sudden and unexplainable death of infants, from birth through one year of age. More boys than girls are victims, and most deaths happen during the fall, winter, and early spring months.

There is little known about this condition, also known as crib death, that claims the lives of 7,000 babies each year, but the SIDS Foundation has made recommendations about how death from SIDS can be made less likely.

Place your baby on her back to sleep on a firm mattress. Infants don't have the head and neck control to maneuver their air space when placed on their tummies, and some research indicates that SIDS is related to rebreathing carbon dioxide. If your baby has a birth defect or has a breathing, heart, or lung condition, or any other special need, talk to your health care provider. While many mothers worry that infants might choke on their spit-up, research does not indicate this to be a threat. There is no increase in suffocation-related deaths because of back sleeping.

Soft mattresses and pillows pose a hazard because they can fold around your baby's mouth and nose. Avoid the use of frilly, overstuffed comforters, sheepskin, heavy fleece, and bumper pads in your baby's crib. If your baby is wearing a sleeper to bed, she needs only a light blanket. Similarly, don't place stuffed animals, toys, or pillows in your baby's cradle. These, too, are suffocation hazards.

Mommy Must

While the exact cause of SIDS is unknown, studies have shown that SIDS deaths are more common in families who smoke. So don't smoke around your baby, and don't allow others to smoke around your baby. Just as you wouldn't smoke in bed for your own health reasons, do not smoke in bed with your baby.

Chapter 6

Am I Doing This Right?

UNLIKE A BOTTLE, YOU can't measure what's in a breast. As a result, many mothers are concerned about their milk supply. They wonder if they might not have enough milk to nourish their infant. This is a common, but unnecessary, fear. Our uncertainty over our milk supply arises because we like to measure everything scientifically. When you breastfeed, there is no reliable direct method of knowing how much milk your baby receives, but doctors generally follow two guidelines when assessing breastmilk intake: infant weight gain and elimination patterns.

Your Baby's Health

You can easily tell if your infant is receiving an adequate milk supply by monitoring weight gain. Keep in mind, it's normal for babies to lose 5 to 8 percent of their birth weight during the first few days of life. After that, babies should gain about one ounce of weight per day, and by their two-week checkup, they should surpass their birth weight by a few ounces.

A baby who weighs less than her birth weight at her two-week checkup might not be feeding adequately.

When looking at a growth chart, keep in mind that breastfed babies gain weight more rapidly than formula-fed infants during the first two months of life, then slow down around the fourth month. By six months of age, their birth weight should have doubled. If you have concerns about your baby's weight, call your doctor. You can have your baby weighed any time.

Elimination Patterns Explain Growth

The second best indicator of adequate milk intake is frequent bowel movements and urination. What goes in must come out.

While your baby's digestive system is still growing and working out the kinks, you will see some strange things in the first couple of days. Soon after birth, your baby will pass meconium, a thick, sticky, dark substance produced by the liver. After two days, the color of your baby's bowel movements will change to a greenish-brown and will look like thick pea soup. He will pass two to three stools per day. By day five, your baby's stools will change again, this time to a

Mommy Knows Best

After weighing your little one, you may learn that your child is at the high or low end of the growth chart; but this shouldn't be too much of a concern. Growth charts were developed using formula-fed infants as the baseline, so don't worry if your baby weighs in lower than "normal" on the chart.

loose, yellow mustard, cottage cheese, or seedlike consistency. These are called milk stools. Your baby will pass two to five stools per day, most likely during a feeding, or when he's fast asleep and ready to be put down.

Your baby will also wet frequently. During the first two days, he might wet only once or twice. The colostrum you produce is highly digestible and perfect nutrition for your baby, so there's not much left to eliminate. After your abundant milk comes in, your baby will wet five to eight cloth diapers per day, or four to six disposables. With the ultra-absorbent diapers on the market, it can be hard to tell how many wet diapers he really has. You can lay a Kleenex inside the diaper to help you tell when your baby urinates.

The urine will be pale yellow or colorless and odorless. If it's dark or looks like redbrick dust, it could be a sign that your baby is not getting enough milk. If your baby is wetting frequently but not stooling, he might not be getting enough hindmilk.

If your baby is not passing at least two stools per day and wetting six to eight diapers after his first week of life, he could be on his way to dehydration. This

Mindful Mommy

There are many signs that can alert you to the fact that your baby is dehydrated. You should call your pediatrician if your baby exhibits the following symptoms of dehydration: lethargy, weak cry, dry mouth, depressed or sunken fontanel (soft spot) on the top of his head, loss of skin resilience (springiness), or fever.

is a very serious health threat for babies. Talk to your pediatrician immediately.

Colic: It's Tough on Everyone

Your baby can express herself in one way, and one way only, when she is little—by crying. And she will quickly learn that crying is powerful! It is your baby's most effective means of communication. Babies cry for many different reasons. They cry when they're hungry. They cry when they're wet or have a dirty diaper. They cry when they feel scared, lonely, or hurt. They even cry when they're bored. Within the first two weeks of life, you'll learn to distinguish between your baby's different cries. You'll even be able to distinguish her cries from others in a roomful of babies!

Whenever your child cries, you know something is wrong and you instinctively come to her aid. Usually, you can find the problem quickly. You pick up your baby, check her diaper, reassure her, and perhaps offer her a breast. When nothing seems to work, laypeople will call it colic. Pediatricians are a little

Mommy Knows Best

While there are many theories, there is no general agreement as to the cause of colic. Studies show that 10 to 15 percent of newborns (and parents) suffer from colic. Symptoms usually begin within a few weeks of birth and last from three to four months.

more precise, but not much. They usually consider a baby to be colicky if she follows the rule of three: She cries continuously for three or more hours, three or more times each week, for three or more weeks.

The word *colic* is really a catchall for any condition that causes inconsolable crying and screaming in infants. Colicky babies are in pain. Often, their tummies are hard and distended. They arch their backs, ball their fists, flail their arms and legs, and have a hard time with everything from nursing to sleeping. Most babies will calm down when put to the breast and fall asleep shortly after feeding, but not a colicky baby. A colicky baby is more likely to suck vigorously for just a few minutes and then pull away screaming and struggling.

Fussiness versus Colic

You may be wondering if your crying baby is just fussy or if he is colicky. Many parents think about this on a daily basis—worrying that it's the latter! But there are ways to tell the difference. Crying infants are difficult to feed and do not breastfeed effectively. Fussy infants can be consoled at the breast. Most colicky infants cannot.

Every baby will have periods of fussiness, especially during the first few weeks of life. Not only are they new to the world, but the world is new to them. It's louder, colder, and brighter than the womb, and it can take some getting used to.

Like adults, every baby has a different temperament, and some are naturally more demanding and sensitive than others. You can think of these high-maintenance babies as having especially sharp senses. Gas pain that wouldn't upset most babies can be very distressing to one with more delicate sensibilities.

Growth Spurts and Your Baby's Feedings

Babies grow in spurts and during these times they are often cranky and confused. Growth spurts usually occur around two to three weeks and again at six weeks. During these times, your baby might fuss because she is hungry. You're making enough milk, it's just time to take production up another notch. Your baby is growing and prepping your body for the additional nourishment she needs.

Babies experiencing growth spurts tend to feed more often, especially during the evening. After several cluster feeds, your baby will doze off for several hours. Because your milk supply is lower in the evening, your baby can cluster feed without developing gastritis.

Letting your baby nurse more often will quickly increase your milk supply and satisfy her appetite. If you are returning to work during this time, frequent pumping is important.

Mindful Mommy

Watch your baby closely to see if she develops crying patterns. You can determine if a crying baby is fussy or if she has colic by doing this. Standard fussiness seems to follow predictable patterns. Crying often peaks with babies in their second week of life. They cry more frequently and with more intensity because of environmental overstimulation and growth spurts.

Causes of Colic

Because no one quite knows what colic is, there's no way to tell for sure what causes it. There are many theories though. Immature digestive and nervous systems are often thought to be at the root of colic simply because babies seem to miraculously grow out of it by four months of age, a time when those systems have become significantly more developed. For some babies, many different factors can come into play.

Allergies

One common theoretical cause of colic is food allergy. Tiny particles of food, called allergens, find their way from your body into your breastmilk. Some of these allergens simply irritate your baby's intestinal lining. Others leak through that lining and enter your baby's bloodstream, causing her immune system to respond. The typical symptoms of a food allergy in infants are rashes, gas, discolored and mucousy stools, vomiting, a stuffy nose, a red ring around the anus, or a refusal to nurse.

GER

Another cause of colic is gastroesophageal reflux, or GER. Basically, GER is a condition in which immature development of a muscular valve at the intersection of the stomach and the esophagus lets stomach acid enter your child's esophagus. The acid causes a painful sensation like heartburn. Babies who spit up a lot and fail to gain weight are often diagnosed with GER. This is a serious condition and must be monitored by your health care provider. Breastfed babies are three times less likely to have GER than formula-fed babies.

The other typical causes of colic have to do with the way your baby nurses. Too much milk let down too quickly causes a baby to take big gulps of air, leading to an upset stomach. Air can also be swallowed if your baby's mouth doesn't form a tight seal around the breast. Some of the latest research on colic and nursing has shown that some babies might become colicky when they switch from breast to breast too soon and fill up on foremilk. Foremilk is very lactose-rich and the excess lactose can ferment in your baby's body, causing gas, bloating, and explosive, greenish stools. This doesn't mean your baby is lactose-intolerant. It just means he's getting too much foremilk.

How Long Will It Last?

Colic is such a tricky condition. You may be lying awake, those sleepless, loud nights, wondering—when will this end? But no one can say with certainty

Mommy Must

When your baby is at your breast, and you hear a frequent clicking or slurping sounds, she may have a poor seal between the breast and her mouth or her tongue is out of position. Poor latch will allow your baby to swallow air, increasing the chances of an upset stomach and gas pains.

how long a baby (and her parents) will suffer from colic. Some babies suffer for months, while others recover in a few days. The same is true regarding the timing and duration of a particular episode of colicky screaming. Some babies cry only at certain times of day, and others scream inconsolably day and night.

Eventually, whatever it is gets better. Most children recover from colic by the beginning of their fourth month of life. Historically, people called colic in newborns "three-month colic," indicating an awareness of that wonderful fourth month. Even food allergies and the heartburn-like pain of GER will pass. By six months of age, your baby's intestines will be mature enough to handle most food proteins that are present in your breastmilk. Within the next six months, the muscular valve at the top of your baby's stomach will have developed enough to prevent GER.

Coping with a Colicky Infant

If you have determined that your little one is not just fussy, and you are sure that colic is the cause of her unrest, there are some things that you can do to ease her stress. Respond quickly to her cries. Offer the breast. Provide any physical security she might need.

If your baby can't be consoled, make an appointment with your pediatrician right away. Doctors typically use a diagnosis of colic when a baby seems healthy and is gaining weight but can't be consoled. Insist that your child's health care provider make a reasonable effort to find the problem.

A diagnosis of GER gives you a chance to reduce both the frequency and the severity of colic attacks. As always, breast is best. Your milk digests more rapidly than formula in your baby's stomach, so there's less chance for stomach contents to back up into the esophagus. Doctors recommend that feedings be frequent and small. Propping up the head of the crib is also helpful in keeping stomach acid down.

A lactation consultant can help you determine if your baby has a good latch by observing a feeding. If it is determined that your baby is swallowing air, there are solutions. Check your nursing posture and the feeding position of your baby, and make her open her mouth wide before you let her take the breast.

If you suspect your baby isn't nursing long enough on each breast to get hindmilk, remember to let her nurse as long as she wants before switching

Mindful Mommy

Talk to your doctor about how to position your baby when she sleeps. Sometimes babies with GER sleep better on their stomachs. But stomach sleeping has been associated with an increased risk of SIDS.

sides. Don't feel that you need to move her to the second breast after some predetermined amount of time. Clocks can't tell you when to switch sides. Both your breasts and your baby will quickly adjust to this change in the feeding pattern.

If your baby seems to quit nursing before your let-down occurs, try breast compression to get her interested again. Breast compression is very much like manual milk expression, except that you do it while your baby still has your breast in her mouth.

What Are You Eating?

After you've eliminated medical causes and nursing problems from your list of suspects, take a look at your diet. Most women can eat anything they want while breastfeeding and never experience any problems. A few of us aren't so lucky.

There are certain foods that seem to cause colic symptoms more than others, but every breastfeeding woman and every nursing child is unique. Consider any list of "problem" foods to be nothing more than a convenient starting point for your tests.

Mindful Mommy
Your child is more likely to be sensitive to stray food proteins if you have a history of food allergies in your family. Some of these food proteins might be showing up in your breastmilk and you'd never know it! You might even be allergic to a food yourself and not realize it.

Problem Foods: The Usual Suspects*

Ingredient	Reaction
Caffeine	Because very young infants can't eliminate caffeine from their bodies very well, it can build up in their system and make them irritable. Caffeine is present in chocolate, soft drinks, coffee, tea, and some cold medicines.
Chocolate	Theobromine, a chemical found in chocolate, irritates the lining of a baby's stomach, resulting in fussiness or diarrhea.
Citrus fruits	Oranges, grapefruits, lemons, and limes can irritate a baby's stomach and intestines. Symptoms include sniffles, diarrhea, skin rashes, fussiness, hives, or vomiting.
Cow's milk	Dairy products are the most common cause of allergic reactions in infants. Symptoms can include cough, diarrhea, fussiness, gas, rash, runny nose, or congestion.
Eggs, wheat, corn, fish, nuts, soy	These foods can pass into your milk and cause diarrhea, skin rashes, hives, sniffles, fussiness, or vomiting
Gassy vegetables	Cauliflower, onion, garlic, cabbage, broccoli, peppers, cucumbers, and turnips can cause gas and fussiness, especially when eaten raw.
Spicy foods	Spicy foods probably cause problems simply by changing the flavor of your milk or, rarely, by irritating your baby's stomach. The only symptom is usually a refusal to nurse.

*Medicines and iron supplements are also commonly blamed for colic.

Once you've identified a food that seems to cause a reaction in your baby, eliminate it from your diet. Most foods will clear from your body within forty-eight hours, but it may be a week or so before the last traces of some foods are gone. During that transitional time, your baby's colic might continue. Hang in there and remember that colic can be caused by a combination of things, so eliminating a problem food can often be just the first step.

Soothing Sounds

As strange as it sounds, your vacuum cleaner is about to become your new best friend. The sound of a vacuum has been known to instantly calm a colicky baby. Get out the Hoover and give it a try. If you can't use the vacuum cleaner, tune the television to a static-filled channel and turn up the volume. Other good sources of white noise are detuned radios or small appliances like blenders and mixers.

Don't underestimate the power of your own voice cooing softly in your baby's ear. Use your voice as an instrument. Sing. Change tones. Babies respond well to "parentese," that higher-pitched tone moms and dads often use when speaking to infants.

Mommy Knows Best

During the stressful and unsettling experience with colicky baby, you might be tempted to just forget about breastfeeding and switch to formula. But stick it out. Most babies who have a food allergy are sensitive to cows' milk, the primary ingredient in baby formula. Instead of eliminating colic, formula may actually make it worse.

Good Vibrations

Movement is soothing to all babies. Anyone who has ever cared for a crying child knows that rocking, bouncing, or the gentle vibrations of a moving vehicle can lull a baby into sleep. Calming movement seems instinctive when you try to soothe your child. Most parents have tried rocking and gently bouncing their baby in their arms, but don't stop there. Try dancing, moving from side to side, baby swings, and bouncy chairs.

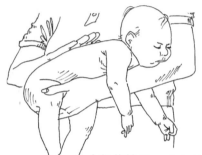

Colic Hold: The colic hold places gentle pressure on your baby's tummy, which may ease digestive pains. Combine this hold with rhythmic motions and soothing sounds to help keep both you and your baby calm.

A variation on the colic hold turns the baby around on your arm (with her head toward your palm) and lets your other arm come up underneath to help support the baby's weight.

Warm Baths Do Wonders

Some parents have found that taking a colicky baby into a tub of warm water will calm her. This is not only great therapy for your child, it's wonderfully relaxing for you. At the first sign of colic, you both get into the bath and stay there. You might be there all morning or half the night. Just keep adding warm water along the way and nursing when you need to. Lay your baby on your chest, tuck her knees to her tummy and cover her with a warm washcloth. Gently and continuously cup warm water over her back. The moist heat and skin-to-skin contact have been known to work wonders. Washing your baby with a gentle, scented cleanser enhances the relaxing effects of the bath with a combination of aromatherapy and massage. Lavender is a calming scent for both of you.

The use of aromatherapy in childhood can lead to a lifetime of relaxation. Nothing brings back a memory like the smells associated with an event. Think about your grandmother's kitchen at Thanksgiving or the smell of a vinyl Barbie doll on Christmas morning. The soft sweetness of the lavender that calms your colicky child now will probably become associated with a feeling of relief and relaxation for the rest of her life.

Mindful Mommy

Although a warm bath can provide a welcome break from the symptoms of colic for your baby, parents need to take extreme caution with this approach. A tired mom or dad in the bath can easily fall asleep and an infant could drown.

Snuggle Up

Swaddling is a way of snugly wrapping your infant in a blanket. This technique sometimes helps to calm a colicky baby. Swaddling keeps her warm and secure, like a cloth hug. It's also a way to keep her from being upset by the way her own body suddenly jerks when she's startled. Swaddled babies often sleep longer and fuss less.

During early infancy, most babies are swaddled from the neck down. Your baby might prefer to have her arms free. Try it both ways. Older babies, however, are generally frustrated by swaddling. If your child is learning to roll or crawl, it's probably time to give up the swaddling.

Slings

Slings act as "transitional wombs." Slings have been used for centuries by people in other cultures to keep their babies close to their bodies for warmth, protection, and transportation. Your baby is close to your breast, can hear your heartbeat, and grows in sync with your body rhythms. Dads who carry their babies in slings bond more quickly as both learn to read each other's cues and movements. Baby-wearing meets an infant's need for sensory stimulation. Constant contact with their caregivers promotes happier, healthier babies, and studies indicate that sling-carried infants cry less frequently than other babies.

Infant Massage

Another great way to help relieve your colicky baby is by massage. It can help your baby's body release trapped gas by pushing gas and fecal matter through the intestines to the bowel. Massage also promotes the normal functioning of the intestines, stimulates nervous system development, and provides an opportunity for mother and child to work together in a relaxing and bonding way.

When massaging your baby, use a light natural oil (like vegetable oil), not lotion. Baby oil has petroleum products that can seep into baby's skin. Keep all of your motions gentle, long, slow, and rhythmic.

A Stressful Time for Mom and Dad

Having a newborn is stressful enough; add to that the fact that she is a colicky baby, and you may feel like there's no way out. The stress caused by a screaming baby, combined with a new parent's lack of confidence and lack of sleep, can take a huge toll on your health and self-esteem. A baby with colic puts a tremendous strain on a family, especially on a nursing mother. It's not uncommon for women to feel disappointed and even angry about their colicky

Mommy Knows Best
There's no such thing as a spoiled infant!

child. Remember that it's not your baby's fault. She's not crying because she is spoiled or greedy. She's simply in pain.

Many colicky babies have their crying jags in the evening when you're already worn out from the day's activities, so sleep whenever you can. Always good advice to new parents, it's incredibly important for parents of a colicky baby. One of you can take the baby to a far corner of the house or on a long drive while the other naps. Fathers need to step up during colic attacks and offer relief to their breastfeeding partners whenever they can.

Over time, the screaming and crying can really wear you and your partner down and deflate your excitement about being parents. Every expectant couple has a dream about what it's going to be like when the baby finally arrives. We all envision an "easy" baby, a baby that's sweet and loving and even fun. The reality is that the arrival of a new baby is a huge change for the entire family. On a scale of one to ten, a "normal" baby changes your life by about nine and a colicky baby changes it by about a thousand. Your colicky baby will get better and things will get easier. Keep reminding yourself and your spouse of that!

Mommy Knows Best

Colic just happens. Don't blame yourself or anyone else! A colicky baby does not make you a bad parent. It also doesn't mean there's anything wrong with your breastmilk or your genetics. There seems to be no common thread connecting colicky infants—not birth order, culture, class, gender, or anything that happened during pregnancy or birth.

When colic threatens to overwhelm you, express a bottle of breastmilk and get away for a while. Give the baby to your partner and go somewhere special, just for you. Remember that colic is only temporary. Your entire family can get through this and move on to the truly wonderful times that lay ahead for all of you.

What Your Infant Needs

Most women produce an ounce of milk per breast per hour. Breasts generally feel full before a feeding and softer afterward, but because breasts don't have fuel gauges, the only surefire way to measure your milk is to express it. Even then, you won't get a true indication of your milk volume. A pump simply cannot remove milk as efficiently as your baby can. Your breasts change during pregnancy, then once more with the birth of your baby, and again after a solid nursing routine is established. Lactogenesis leaves breasts full within three to five days postpartum.

According to infant studies, your baby needs about one to two ounces of milk per feeding per month of age.

Day 1: 5 ccs (colostrum)
Day 2: 15 ccs or ½ ounce (colostrum)
Day 3: 30 ccs or 1 ounce (colostrum)
Day 4: 2 ounces (transitional milk)
Day 5: 2–2½ ounces (transitional milk)

You can also gauge how much your baby needs at each feeding by his weight:

6–8 pounds:	2 ounces
9–12 pounds:	3 ounces
13–15 pounds:	4 ounces
15+ pounds:	5 ounces

As your baby suckles, you might feel a tingling or pins-and-needles sensation that lets you know your milk is letting down. As you nurse your baby, milk leaking from the opposite breast is also a sign that your milk has letdown.

Some women don't have these sensations, nor do they observe leakage. If you don't know if your milk has letdown, you might need the assistance of a lactation consultant. Stress and fatigue can inhibit the milk ejection reflex, and this can ultimately reduce your milk supply.

Some mothers feel tenderness during their first week of breastfeeding. However, this discomfort usually subsides after the baby has latched on correctly. If you experience sore, cracked, or blistered nipples,

Mommy Knows Best

If you've had an epidural during labor, talk to a lactation consultant before hospital discharge, as you may be overhydrated. Epidurals often cause overhydration of body tissues, which in turn makes it difficult for hormones that stimulate the production of milk, like prolactin, to reach breast cells across this lake of fluid.

your baby is not latching on correctly and might not be adequately removing milk from the breast.

If you have not experienced any change in your breasts during pregnancy or after the birth of your baby, you'll need to have a breast exam performed by your doctor. A rare condition exists in a very few women that affects the growth of their mammary tissues. This underdevelopment inhibits milk production. Women who have had breast reduction surgery or a mastectomy are also at risk for insufficient milk production. If your doctor has determined that you are physically incapable of producing enough milk to nourish your baby, you might be asked to supplement with formula.

Supplemental Feeding and Alternative Methods

After consulting with your doctor or lactation consultant, and determining that your baby isn't getting enough milk, you can all work together to increase your milk production. There are many things that you can do, in fact, that will help you produce more milk. Some strategies to increase your prolactin levels and help you produce a more abundant supply are:

- Increase breastfeeding frequency
- Feed from both breasts
- Express your breastmilk with a double pump

There may be situations that require you to use an alternative feeding method for a short time as you build your milk supply. With the goal of exclusive breastfeeding in mind, practice any of these methods cautiously and only under the guidance of a lactation consultant or pediatrician. Alternative feeding should be used on a temporary basis to correct breastfeeding problems. It's not usually a viable long-term solution, and it's important to get your baby back to the breast as soon as possible.

Supplemental Feeding Devices and Techniques

Type: Cup Feeding
Description: A flexible one- or two-ounce cup is filled with milk and held to baby's lips. The baby is held upright and allowed to lick at the milk.
Comments: DO NOT POUR. Baby should not be crying at start.

Type: Spoon Feeding
Description: This method is similar to cup feeding but utilizes a spoon. A small, soft spoon is best. Some special spoons hold larger amounts of milk in a reservoir so feeding isn't interrupted.
Comments: Tedious and time-consuming but effective.

Type: Syringe or Eyedropper Feeding
Description: An eyedropper can be used to drip milk into an upright baby's mouth. A syringe can be used in the same way. A syringe with a long tip can be used to feed at the breast.
Comments: Periodontal syringes are best; they have a soft tip that won't hurt baby's gums.

Type: Finger Feeding
Description: The tube of a supplemental feeder is held to a clean adult finger. Baby sucks on the finger and gets milk through the tube.
Comments: Effective but some babies prefer it to the breast.

Type: Supplemental Nutrition System
Description: A supplemental nutrition system is used when baby can latch onto the breast but needs supplemental feeding. Typically, a reservoir of milk is worn around the mom's neck and tubes from it are inserted into baby's mouth as he suckles. Baby gets both milks—from the breast and from the supplementer.
Comments: #1 recommended method. Builds Mom's morale. Teaches proper latch on and stimulates milk production.

Type: Haberman Feeder
Description: A special bottle with a long nipple and a valve that rewards any level of suckling.
Comments: Useful for babies with developmental delays or oral/facial abnormalities.

Type: Standard Bottle
Description: Any variety of the plain old infant bottle.
Comments: May lead to nipple confusion and poor suck.

Figuring Out Supplemental Systems

Supplemental nursing systems, like Medela's SNS or Lact-Aid International's Nursing Trainer, consist of a milk reservoir and a short length of very small, clear tubing. The reservoir is worn around a mother's neck from a cord and the tubing is inserted into the baby's mouth as he nurses at the breast. This technique is the method of choice for most lactation professionals as it allows the breast to be stimulated to increase milk production, helps infants learn proper latch, and preserves the breastfeeding relationship.

Supplementers are used with infants who have weak sucks or nipple confusion from supplemental bottle feeding in the hospital. It's also beneficial for mothers who suffer from reduced milk supply.

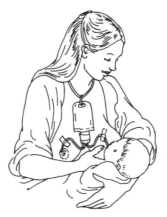

A Supplemental Nutrition System: These systems supplement your baby's feeding while you continue to breastfeed.

You can make your own supplementer by cutting a hole in the nipple of a bottle. Add expressed milk or formula. Place one end of a small gavage tube (available at a medical supply store) into the hole. Position your baby at your breast in the cradle or football hold. As you support your breast in the C hold, tuck the tube under your thumb, extending it toward the end of your nipple. Latch your baby to your breast and the tube.

As your infant suckles, he not only receives the milk from the reservoir, but he stimulates and extracts milk from your breast at the same time. Carefully adjust the flow rate to match your baby's ability to keep up. You should be able to hear him swallow milk, but the flow should never be fast enough to cause gagging.

Cup or Spoon Feeding

Another way to feed your baby is by using a cup or a spoon. Liquid dispelled in this way can be beneficial for a baby who has jaundice, poor elimination patterns, or inadequate latch. Cup feeding reduces nipple confusion from a bottle and allows the infant to lap milk at his own pace. It can be messy, but it's an easy substitution for breastfeeding.

To begin, place a towel around your baby or swaddle him in a blanket. Fill a spoon or a soft, flexible cup half full with expressed milk. Bring the cup or spoon to the baby's lower lip. Drip just enough milk into his mouth to taste. Tip the spoon so your baby can lick the milk. This process is slower than putting baby to the breast but can be used to supplement breastfeeding, as needed. Use of a well-cleaned eyedropper can also be effective.

Finger Feeding:
Not Easy, But Helpful

Finger feeding is hard to learn, is awkward, and can cause dependency, but it is useful for babies who have a weak suck, nipple confusion, or neurological problems.

Insert a small gavage tube into the nipple of a baby bottle filled with expressed milk. Place your baby in a semi-reclining position. Place a clean finger (nail side down) slowly into your baby's mouth, moving it back to the soft palate. If your baby gags, bring your finger forward slightly, and wait until he's comfortable. Place the tube or periodontal syringe next to your finger. As your baby suckles, he will draw milk from the bottle, or you can offer a small squirt from the syringe.

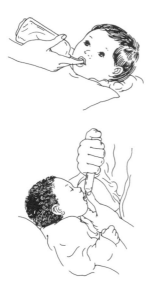

Finger Feeding: This alternative method uses expressed milk and allows your baby to suck on your finger, rather than a nipple.

Syringe Feeding: Like finger feeding, syringe feeding delivers expressed milk when feeding at the breast is not possible.

A Last Resort: Bottle Feeding

Bottle feeding might be the only alternative available when other techniques don't work. It can be useful for mothers with sore nipples or if an infant can't open his mouth wide enough to latch to the breast. However, many babies who switch from breast to bottle and back again will suffer from nipple confusion. Bottle nipples flow faster than the breast, and once babies develop a dependency on the bottle, they often refuse the breast.

Many parents find that infants accept supplemental feedings more easily from Dad than from Mom. A baby grows comfortable with the breast-feeding relationship she establishes with her mother and can sometimes be confused when her breastfeeding buddy tries to offer a less satisfying alternative. Supplemental and alternative feeding methods give Dad a wonderful opportunity to take part in the feeding of his child. Finger feeding, cup feeding, spoons, bottles, and eyedroppers can be used by anyone. Many fathers enjoy being able to solve problems, and giving supplemental feedings can be a rewarding way to help them feel more connected to their children.

Mindful Mommy

Supplemental feedings are meant to be just that, supplemental! If you decide to use formula again and again, your milk supply will quickly diminish. Early use of a bottle can even delay your milk from coming in. Use supplemental bottle feeding with caution: It can quickly end the breastfeeding relationship.

Chapter 7

Is This Normal?

IT IS ENTIRELY NORMAL to wonder: is this normal? While breastfeeding and throughout life, there are challenges that you will face with uncertainty and anxiety. Whether your baby has difficulty latching on or you need to suspend breastfeeding for your own health reasons, anything that interferes with milk removal can diminish your supply. If your baby doesn't take in enough milk, your body won't produce enough milk. Fortunately, most breastfeeding problems are easily resolved if you catch them early enough.

Painful Problems

While you and your baby are learning to breastfeed together, you may experience some temporary discomfort the first week or so. Your baby takes your nipple and part of the areola to the back of his mouth, and he compresses the areola to express milk from the sinuses. You should feel a gentle tug that will take some getting used to.

If you do feel actual nipple pain while nursing, your baby might not be positioned correctly. Your nipple has more pain receptors than your areola, so, if your baby is feeding from the nipple, you'll feel it. Continued nipple feeding can lead to cracked or blistered nipples. Break the latch and try again. If everything else seems to be all right but nipple pain persists after a week, check for thrush.

You might feel some minor breast discomfort with your milk ejection reflex or letdown. Sensations vary from slight tingles to pins and needles. Letdown lasts less than thirty seconds. You'll also feel some breast fullness with engorgement; however, this normally decreases within two days.

Is It Engorgement?

It just sounds painful doesn't it? What is it? Why does it happen? When? Engorgement usually happens around three to five days postpartum. Your mature milk comes in, in preparation for exclusive breast-feeding. When engorgement happens, it can be extremely uncomfortable. You wake up one morning

Mommy Must

As every new mother is aware of every little change in her baby, make sure to evaluate the way that you are feeling too! If you have prolonged nipple pain, there could be something wrong. Contact your lactation consultant for help.

with breasts the size of cantaloupes. They're swollen, your nipple and areola are tight, and your baby has little flexible tissue to latch onto. While this lasts only for a couple of days, it can be painful.

Frequent feedings will help reduce engorgement. They will also regulate your milk supply. If your baby has difficulty latching on, express just enough milk to make yourself comfortable and your breasts pliable. After your baby has had her fill, you can express more milk and either refrigerate or freeze it for later use. (Remember, though, that any milk that is removed will be replaced. That's the law of supply and demand.)

Warm showers will relieve the pressure of engorgement, and your milk will begin to leak naturally. Heat, in general, will soften your breasts. A warm washcloth on full breasts can help to alleviate discomfort.

Cabbage Leaves—A Curious Remedy

For one reason or another, cabbage leaves seem to help relieve pain due to engorgement. Although there is no known medical reason why cabbage leaves should help with engorgement, many mothers and lactation professionals will attest to the fact that

Mommy Knows Best
Only use cabbage leaves as long as the engorgement lasts. If you use them for longer, you can inadvertently diminish your milk supply.

they work. Cabbage leaves have been used through-out the centuries in other countries. It's a timeless, yet "new age," method for reducing engorgement.

So how can you prepare these leaves for yourself and your poor breasts? First, buy a medium cabbage and peel and clean the leaves. Store them in Ziploc bags. Refrigerate. When you're ready to use them, select enough leaves to completely cover your breasts on all sides, as well as the area under your armpit. Gently crush the leaves to break the veins, then apply the cool leaves to your breasts. Lie back on a towel and relax, or tuck them securely into your bra. The cool cabbage leaves will help reduce the pain and swelling associated with engorgement.

Within two hours, you should begin to feel relief. Some milk might leak, so if you're using the bra method, line your bra with nursing pads or other absorbent materials. You should reapply new leaves after two hours, or whenever they appear wilted.

Other Techniques to Alleviate Pain

Although the engorgement phase is relatively brief, you'll want to give yourself every advantage to ensure your comfort until your nursing routine is established. In addition to cool cabbage leaves and warm showers, consider the following suggestions:

- Take ibuprofen (Motrin, Nuprin, or Advil) for pain.

- Wear a supportive bra.
- Wrap a plastic bag of ice chips or frozen vegetables in a washcloth. (Peas or corn work best because of their size, but you can use whatever is available.) The bag will conform to the shape of your breast and can be used for fifteen to twenty minutes of relief. If you plan to refreeze the bag of vegetables and use it again later, mark it as inedible. Repeated freezing and thawing promotes the growth of bacteria.
- A refrigerated rice sock works wonders, too. Rice socks are used by doulas to relieve pain during labor. They conform to your body and provide relief by interrupting the pain receptors that carry messages to the brain. Rice socks can be heated or cooled. To cool, toss it in the freezer for an hour. To heat, toss it in the microwave for thirty seconds at a time (for up to two minutes). When using the microwave method, carefully shake the sock so the heat is evenly distributed. Wrap the rice sock in a washcloth or sheet to protect your skin.

Remember that this stage is only temporary. Try any combination of the relief methods until the discomfort passes and you and your baby can have a comfortable breastfeeding session.

Learn about Leaking

It is common to worry about a leaking nipple and unfortunately it is a common occurrence too! While it can happen, some lucky women don't experience any leaking at all. Leaking most often occurs during the first few weeks of lactation and usually only continues with women who have a very abundant milk supply. There are exceptions, of course, and leaking or even spraying milk during lovemaking is common.

If you experience frequent leaking:

- Nurse your baby frequently, especially before going out or making love.
- Use absorbent cotton breastpads or cloths to catch the drips.
- Place bath towels under you when in bed.
- Press your folded arms gently against your chest to draw your breasts into your body.

There are occasions when you'll experience letdown at the thought or smell of your baby. A crying child in the supermarket might even turn on your milk like a faucet. Generally, though, most women who feed their babies regularly won't leak after a breastfeeding routine is well established.

Sore Nipples and Blisters

Cracked, sore, and blistered nipples are signs of improper latch. All of these things are very unpleasant and painful! When babies feed only on the nipple, nipples can crack and blister. Blisters also occur as a result of the nipple rubbing against the roof of baby's mouth or along his gums. The pain associated with a blistered nipple can make nursing very uncomfortable, but it's important to continue breastfeeding.

Sometimes cracked nipples bleed, but that doesn't have to interfere with nursing. A little bit of your blood, mixed with your milk, will not harm your baby.

First, you should consult your lactation consultant to set up an appointment. He or she will watch a nursing session with you and your baby and will instruct you both how to make the feeding successful. In the meantime, to treat sore nipples:

- Ensure that your baby has a good latch. (Wait until he opens wide, then grasp him to the breast, pointing your nipple to the roof of his mouth. He needs to take in an inch of the areola as well.)
- Use different nursing positions to vary the way your baby latches onto your nipple.
- Offer the least tender breast first so that your milk will let down in the other breast without your baby creating suction.

- Express your milk using a pump to help your milk let down before offering your breast to your baby.
- Break suction evenly by inserting your finger into your baby's mouth. (Don't allow your baby to slide off your nipple.)
- Apply lanolin to a sore nipple. (Like chapped lips, nipples heal more quickly with moisture. You don't need to remove modified lanolin before your baby nurses.)
- Use breast shells to keep your nipples from rubbing against fabric.

Remember, also, to avoid using soap on your nipples. The Montgomery glands produce natural oils to clean and protect your nipples; soap may aggravate the situation by drying them out further.

Plugged Ducts

Another painful experience that some mothers face is a plugged duct. This occurs when there is an insufficient removal of milk from the breast. The retained milk forms a cheeselike blockage in the duct, causing a small lump that might be painful, red, or swollen. If neglected, plugged ducts can lead to infections.

The best way to prevent a plugged duct is simply to breastfeed as often as your baby wants, making sure that he finishes one breast before starting another. It's also helpful to change nursing positions. Different positions help your baby remove the milk from all of the ducts. Finally, be sure to wear a comfortable bra. Avoid anything that binds or constrains the breasts, including underwires.

If one of your ducts does become plugged, check for a plugged nipple. Milk residue can sometimes dry in a nipple pore, forming a blockage. If you see a small white dot, like a whitehead, on your nipple, you might have a plugged pore. Nipple blockages are often removed by your baby's suckling. They can also be removed by your health care provider, although many women find that careful work with a fingernail does the trick.

If no nipple blockage is apparent:

- Apply a warm cloth to the affected area for fifteen to twenty minutes before each feeding.
- Nurse more frequently, beginning each session with the affected breast.
- Massage the breast near the plugged duct as your baby nurses or in a warm shower, gently working from behind the plug toward the nipple.

When the plug breaks loose, you might see a filament of solidified milk. It looks like a string and can be several inches in length. If you see one of these strings in your baby's mouth after nursing, don't be alarmed. It's soft and safe to eat, and it won't choke your baby.

The Meaning of Mastitis

It is possible that one or both of your breasts become infected. This type of infection is called mastitis. The infections are bacterial and usually occur as a result of a plugged duct or cracked nipple. You may have mastitis if you have flu-like symptoms along with a fever and a hard spot or lump in the breast accompanied by pain, redness, and swelling. Mastitis is often treated with antibiotics. Other measures include warm showers, lots of bed rest and fluids, and frequent nursing. The infection is not harmful to babies and is only aggravated by weaning.

Anytime mastitis symptoms last beyond two days or a breast lump remains, you should suspect an abscess. A breast abscess is a pool of pus within the breast tissue. The fluid must be drained by your doctor. Recovery is rapid after draining, but temporary weaning from the infected breast might be required.

Thrush

Thrush or candida is another name for a common yeast infection of both mothers and babies. Most children with candida became infected as they passed through the birth canal. The first symptoms usually occur in two to four weeks. On occasion, babies become infected much later, usually after the use of antibiotics. If you've nursed comfortably for many weeks or months but are suddenly experiencing pain, thrush might be the problem.

Thrush can be very painful, but it responds well to treatment. Doctors typically prescribe an antifungal rinse for baby's mouth and an antifungal cream or ointment for baby's bottom (boy or girl) and mother's nipples. However, medication alone is not always effective. In addition to medical treatment, you should:

- Rinse the affected breasts and diaper area with clean water and let them air dry.
- Expose the affected area to the sun for a few minutes, once or twice per day.
- Change your nursing pads after every feeding session.
- Change diapers frequently—yeast thrives in warm, damp places.
- Wash bras, bottle nipples, breast shells, pacifiers, and any other items that come into contact with the infected areas in hot, soapy water.
- Use lanolin or other breastfeeding-friendly nipple treatments to relieve pain.

Mindful Mommy

Infants with thrush have white patches inside their mouths or an angry rash on their bottoms. Mothers often have sharp, shooting pains in their breasts, and sometimes red, tender nipples or patches of red or white on the breast

- Wash your hands before and after each feeding or treatment.
- Drink more water and eat less sugar.
- Treat your partner if he has had contact with your breasts.

Many mothers successfully treat thrush with a nonprescription medication called gentian violet. Most pharmacies carry a 1 percent solution of gentian violet that can be applied to all infected areas with a cotton swab, twice daily for three days. It's a pretty color, but it stains everything it comes in contact with, so be careful with your clothing.

If you are expressing milk while you have a yeast infection, pump and dump. Freezing does not kill yeast and stored milk can re-infect your baby.

Nipple Here, There, Everywhere

Your baby is just getting used to the world around him and he will inevitably look for consistency in an attempt to figure things out. If your baby has been fed from a bottle, he might find it difficult to feed from the breast. Similarly, a baby who's been exclusively breastfed can find the transition to a bottle difficult. Feeding from a bottle is different from breastfeeding. The suck is different. The volume and flow of milk is different. The taste, texture, and temperature are different. Perhaps most importantly, bottles reward lazy nursing and breasts don't.

When your baby doesn't know how to suckle the breast properly because of bottle or pacifier use, it's called nipple confusion. Nipple confusion threatens your breastfeeding success by compromising your milk production. Your infant's disorganized suck won't effectively remove the milk from your breast. That leads to a decreased milk supply, which leads many moms to supplement nursings with a bottle of formula. However, you need a hungry baby's eager suckling to maintain your milk production.

Whether you're transitioning your child from breast to bottle or bottle to breast, be patient and persistent. Your baby will make the change, but it might not happen on the first attempt. The best time to try a new feeding method is when your baby is awake and alert but not too hungry. Your baby will only be frustrated by the change if he's already fussing for dinner. The quiet-alert stage right after he wakes is best.

If you're going from bottle to breast, express some milk before you begin to trigger your letdown reflex. Babies who are used to bottles want their milk immediately. After your baby has caught on to breastfeeding, you can continue nursing him without any special preparation.

Mommy Must

To avoid nipple confusion, simply try to stay away from using bottles! Because nipple confusion impairs breastfeeding success, new moms should avoid giving their infants bottles or pacifiers for at least the first six weeks of life.

If you're transitioning from the breast to a bottle, you might need to experiment with a number of different nipple styles and materials to find one your child likes. There are quite a few varieties available, and babies definitely do have individual preferences. Start the move to bottle feeding with expressed breastmilk, but let Dad or another caregiver do the feeding. Some babies simply refuse to take a bottle from Mom when they know there's a perfectly good breast available.

Breastmilk and Jaundice

Unlike newborn jaundice, breastmilk jaundice usually occurs in well-fed babies who are older than seven days, and it can persist for many weeks. Some doctors believe that breastmilk contains an unknown substance that lets babies absorb an excessive amount of bilirubin, but don't let that theory scare you.

There is nothing wrong with your milk. The usual course of treatment is to monitor your baby's blood and wait for this normal, physiological process to end. Nurse often. Your baby's body eliminates

Mommy Knows Best

If you have been instructed to give your baby formula, pumping your breasts frequently will maintain your milk supply. Ask your doctor about finger feeding or other methods to help reduce nipple confusion while your baby takes formula.

bilirubin in her stools. The greater the frequency of bowel movements, the quicker the excess bilirubin leaves the body.

If phototherapy is advised, use a bilirubin blanket. These blankets have fiber-optic lights built in so you can hold and nurse your baby while she receives her treatment. Occasionally, doctors recommend that a child be given formula instead of breastmilk for twelve to twenty-four hours. This quickly lowers the bilirubin levels in baby's bloodstream. However, even one day of bottle feeding can interfere with your breastfeeding success.

Teething and Biting—Ouch!

You should talk to and reprimand your baby if and when she bites your nipple. She will learn from the tone of your voice that it is wrong to bite you. Tell her "No" and break the latch. Look her in the eye and tell her "No biting." Be serious but not angry. She may already be in tears after your surprised reaction. Offer the breast again, but if she continues to bite, give her a teething toy to help reinforce its use. Offer expressed

Mommy Must

Beware of foods that are choking hazards, like frozen foods, raw vegetables, and hard fruits. Wait until your baby has lots of strong teeth to chew these foods.

milk, water, or juice in a sippy cup to complete the feeding and try breastfeeding again later. Soon, your baby will begin to associate biting with the items you have offered, but your consistency is key.

Luckily, teething begins around six months of age (depending in part on heredity), so most babies are beginning solids. However, some babies are born with a tooth, called a milk tooth, so learning to get around this little dental ditty happens much earlier.

What if your baby refuses the breast because of teething pain? Again, try the cup. Or call your pediatrician about using an over-the-counter infant teething gel. Your little darling might accept the breast more readily if her gums are numbed. You want to ensure that she's receiving adequate nutrition, so offer chilled mashed bananas, expressed breastmilk, or cold 100 percent natural, unsweetened applesauce.

Find the Support You Need

There are many reasons why women quit breastfeeding. Some feel as if they can't produce enough milk, others are too nervous and everyone hears horror stories from their friends. But you should know that, most of the time, the real cause in these cases was a lack of confidence and support.

New moms who aren't sure their baby is getting enough milk through nursing might be tempted to use formula. However, your breasts make only enough milk to supply your baby's demands. If you worry that you're not producing enough milk and offer formula, the amount of milk you produce decreases from a lack of demand. Then, you're in a downward spiral. Less milk means more formula, which means less demand until, pretty soon, you've shut down altogether—all from lack of confidence.

A good lactation consultant or pediatrician can help you be successful. So can your husband, family, and friends. Unfortunately, there will be people who aren't supportive of your decision to breastfeed and they can undermine your breastfeeding experience. Sometimes husbands aren't too thrilled about sharing your breasts with a baby. Even other women might be defensive about your decision to breastfeed, especially if they bottle-fed their own children. This might include your own mother or mother-in-law. When you talk about the virtues of breastfeeding, they might feel a need to justify bottle-feeding. Try to keep their feelings in mind when they criticize your decision to nurse.

Mindful Mommy

Treat others like you hope to be treated. Reassure bottle-feeding moms that they are good mothers, but if nothing works with the critics, surround yourself with positive voices instead. Get together with women who nursed successfully or join a lactation support group. Remember, you can do it!

Chapter 8

What about Pumps and Bottles?

WHETHER YOU'RE RETURNING TO work, relieving engorgement, or pumping milk so you can have a night out, at some point all nursing mothers need to learn the art of expression. Madonna did it. So did Celine Dion, Cindy Crawford, Anita Baker, Andie McDowell, Demi Moore, Faith Hill, Goldie Hawn, Lisa Kudrow, and Heather Locklear. They were all nursing moms who breastfed and expressed milk for their babies.

Pump It Up!

Nothing is as effective in removing milk from your breasts as a baby—not even a breast pump. But you should learn to use one, in any case. It is important to establish a consistent routine of pumping to maintain your supply. The more frequently you pump, the stronger your supply will be, the same way frequent nursing works with your baby.

A New Routine

An easy way to increase your milk production and get into a routine is to begin to express your milk about two weeks before returning to work. You'll want to express about the same time as your baby would naturally nurse each day, or about every two to three hours in a twenty-four-hour period.

Begin pumping for fifteen minutes using a double pump, or thirty minutes using a single pump (fifteen minutes on each side).

You might notice that not much milk is expressed the first few times you try. It takes time for your body to get used to this artificial suction device. It also takes time for your milk to let down. Eventually, you'll notice steady streams and bona fide long-distance sprays from your nipples, but for now, don't worry. Any milk you express is important for your baby's growth. After about a week, you should be able to pump twenty-five ounces or more per day.

When to Pump? When Not to Pump?

If you express your milk in the morning, you will have greater volume. This is because your prolactin levels fluctuate throughout the day—they are lowest

Mommy Knows Best

Milk will come out of your breasts in spurts. But if you watch closely, you will notice that your breasts have their own general flow pattern. Your breasts will start dripping, then squirt, then drip, then slow to a stop. Continue to pump until the milk stops flowing or dripping.

in the evening and highest in the morning. So pump before you wake your baby. You can still nurse her because your breasts are never really empty. Pump again one and a half to two hours later.

The key is to relax! When you're relaxed, milk flows easily. If you have difficulty with letdown when you pump, nurse your baby on one breast while pumping the other. Once your baby engages your milk ejection reflex, your milk will flow more freely.

Manual Expression

Many mothers find that they need to express their milk for other reasons. There will be times when you need to manually express your milk to ensure that your little one is getting enough. Particularly if you are engorged, your baby might have a difficult time finding enough nipple to take into her mouth. You might need to manually express some milk to relieve the fullness in your breasts and provide some elasticity to your nipple and areola.

Manual expression is the least expensive kind of "pumping." It can be easy with practice, but it can be difficult to learn. If done incorrectly, it can cause bruising, tissue damage, or chafed skin. Ask a lactation consultant or health care provider to demonstrate the correct technique. Seeing it in action is different than reading about it in a book. Practice manual expression even if you don't intend to make it a daily routine. At some point you might need to express your milk without the use of a pump.

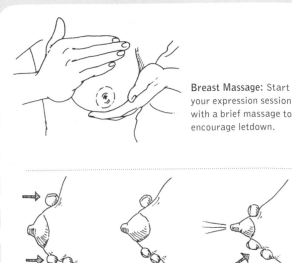

Breast Massage: Start your expression session with a brief massage to encourage letdown.

Manual Expression: This technique requires patience and practice. Remember to rotate as you express to empty all the sinuses.

The How-To's of Manual Expression

1. Wash your hands and gather a clean collection container. A wide-mouth cup strategically placed in front of the nipple will catch your milk as it squirts. Some mothers place a funnel inside a baby bottle to collect their milk.

2. Gently massage your breasts. Use small circular motions as if you're conducting a breast self-exam, or you can do whatever feels comfortable. Start on the outside of the breast and move toward the areola. Bend over at the waist and let gravity assist you. The key is to relax

and allow letdown to occur. Warm washcloths applied to the breast will also help.

3. Place your thumb and first two fingers about one inch behind the nipple or on the edge of the areola in a twelve o'clock and six o'clock position. Your fingers will resemble the letter C.

4. Lift your breast and push it back toward your ribcage.

5. Press down toward the nipple in a gently rolling motion to compress milk out of the sinuses, the way your baby does when she nurses. Don't squeeze the nipple, just the sinuses under the areola. Release your hold and do this again.

6. When milk begins to slow, rotate your hand position around the breast (i.e., eleven and five o'clock) and continue until the sinuses are empty. Work all sides of the breast until milk no longer flows or drips.

7. Rub excess milk onto your nipple and areola.

Eventually, you can try the two-handed, double-breasted method while sitting at a table and expressing milk into a large pan.

Smart Mommy

If you don't intend to store your milk for later, you can also express your milk in a warm shower.

Which Breast Pump Is Right for You?

Every woman is different and it is important to find the breast pump that is right for you! If you intend to express your milk on a regular basis, you'll want to choose a breast pump that meets your individual needs. Criteria vary from person to person, and even over time for the individual. Keep your ultimate goal (whatever it may be) in mind while you shop, and consult your doctor or lactation consultant.

- How often will you use a pump: daily, weekly, or as needed? Are you returning to work or just planning to express an occasional bottle for date night?
- What can you afford? Is this an investment that you intend to use again with other babies or would it be more economical for you to rent?
- Will you be transporting your breast pump to work? Will you need a cooler or carrying case to transport milk back home?
- Will you be expressing in your car?
- What are your power resources?
- How much time do you have to express your milk?
- What kinds of accessories will you need?

When choosing a pump, select the one that most closely imitates your baby's suckling pattern. Pumps that offer the most cycling per minute are the best.

Look for pumps that offer thirty-four to fifty cycles per minute. That timing is most like your baby's nursing pattern. You also want a pump with adjustable suction rates.

In the selection of a breast pump, you truly get what you pay for. Better pumps will cost more, but they express more milk in a shorter period of time, are more comfortable to use, and are less likely to cause tissue damage.

Contact a lactation consultant or certified breastfeeding educator about the different pumps available. They'll share the pros and cons of each model with you and can give you additional information about where to purchase or rent a quality pump. You can also contact your local WIC office, a lactation consultant or breastfeeding educator, or your local birthing center for additional information and recommendations.

Types of Breast Pumps

It's important to choose a reputable brand. These manufacturers have years of experience and a solid history behind their products. A breast pump is an important tool, not a toy. You wouldn't go to a seafood place if you wanted steak, so don't buy a breast pump from a company that specializes in something else.

Check out breast pumps in consumer product safety reports. It's a handy way to compare products based on durability, repair frequency, cost, and any other criteria that are important to you. It's also the place to find out about safety notices and recalls.

Bicycle Horn Pump

Shaped like a bicycle horn, these pumps are the least expensive, but they're also the least effective. You create suction by squeezing and releasing the bulb. Milk is collected into the bulb or a depression in the bottom of the horn. However, because the bulbs can't always be disassembled and cleaned, they can become contaminated with bacterial growth. In addition, bicycle horn pumps can cause breast tissue damage. Unless you are pumping and dumping, this is one to avoid.

Hand- or Foot-Operated Pumps

There are several hand pumps on the market and making a decision about the right one is a difficult task. Most hand pumps offer cylinder-style action or handgrip operation. With cylinder pumps you pull on a piston or plunger to create suction. The flange (a funnel-like contraption) is centered over your nipple. You push the plunger in, then pull it out to draw milk from the breast sinuses.

Hand-grip pumps work in much the same way. They provide suction through the squeeze of a bar. These offer convenient one-handed operation.

Foot-pedal pumps are basically manual pumps that you work with your feet. A hose runs from the pedal to the flange. Foot-pedal pumps offer double pumping, which is the most effective method of expression.

Each of the manual breast pumps is effective and offers good exercise, but they might wear you out. They are best for occasional use only.

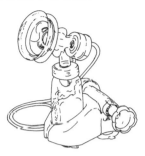

Manual Pump:
Medela Manualectric
Breastpump System

Handheld Battery-Operated Pumps

Battery-operated pumps use a small motor to produce suction. Older pumps require you to manually release the suction, while newer models offer automatic or button suction-release. The motor creates a vacuum on your nipple/areola and you break suction to create the pseudo-nursing effect. Some pumps offer an automatic release that cycles around four to eight times per minute.

Although handheld battery-operated pumps are affordable, they are not very efficient and can cause tissue damage. They're generally slower to create and release suction, so their action doesn't mimic your baby's suckling. In fact, they're often responsible for a diminished milk supply. Many of these pumps are poorly constructed and seem to break just after their ninety-day warranty expires. In addition, they can be noisy and require frequent battery replacement. They are best used for occasional pumping only.

Portable Electric Pumps

These pumps are durable and easy to transport, but often don't offer the optimum number of suction-release cycles. Like many handheld battery-operated machines, some electric pumps depend on the user to break suction. Portable electric pumps often come with accessory packages that offer cigarette lighter adaptors for use in your automobile. They are more effective if you have an abundant milk supply. They also have adjustable suction rates.

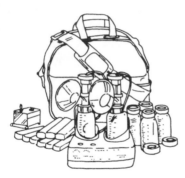

Medela Pump in Style: Even hospital-grade pumps come in a range of sizes and features. Consider whether you will need accessories such as thermal totebags or manual converters.

Hospital-Grade Pumps

These are simply the best and most efficient pumps around. Although they can be expensive to purchase, most hospitals offer rental options for women who intend to pump frequently. Hospital-grade pumps come in several sizes and weights. Some are as light as four pounds while others weigh up to twenty pounds. The lightweight pumps are easily transported and come with adaptors for automobile use.

Look for a pump that provides an automatic suction-release cycle that mimics your baby's suck. Most cycle around forty-eight to sixty times per minute. These pumps offer double pumping, are great for establishing a strong milk supply, and are perfect for the working mother or for use when you have a hospitalized infant. Sometimes hospital-grade pumps are covered by insurance, particularly if your baby is premature or has a medical condition. Suzanne's doctor simply wrote a letter to the insurance company about the benefits of breastfeeding a low-birthweight infant, and they covered all pump expenses for six months. Hospital-grade pumps are most effective and cost-efficient if you use them on a daily basis. Rental fees range from one to three dollars per day.

Pump Process (Twenty to Thirty minutes):

1. Wash your hands with soap and water.
2. Wash all breast pump equipment and assemble it according to the manufacturer's directions.
3. Find a comfortable location to express, just as you would to nurse your baby.
4. Gently massage your breasts or apply a warm washcloth.
5. Center the nipple in the plastic flange. If you are using an electric or battery-operated pump, turn it on the lowest/slowest setting first and increase the speed to match your baby's suck. If you're using a cylinder pump, pull the piston away from your breast, push it back in,

and pull it out again. Try to mimic one suck per second.

6a. Pump the first breast for about seven minutes. (If you are using a double pump, note that you'll follow the pump-massage-pump procedure without switching breasts.)

6b. Switch sides and pump the second breast for seven minutes.

7. Massage your breasts a second time.

8. Return to the first breast for five to seven minutes or until milk no longer flows, followed by the second breast for the same amount of time.

Note: You might have to exchange containers midway through your expression session if your collection bottle becomes full.

9. When milk stops dripping, release suction at the breast as you would with your infant.

10. When you're finished, rub any excess milk onto your nipples and areola.

Mindful Mommy

Make sure that your breast pump fits. You can do this by watching how your nipple enters and exits the flange. If your nipple is squashed, you might need a larger flange neck. Nipples should not rub or touch the sides.

11. Pour the milk into a clean container for storage, or, if a lid is provided with your pump, screw it on tightly.
12. Label the container with the date and the amount, and immediately refrigerate what you don't plan to use within eight to ten hours.
13. Detach the pump and disassemble any washable components. Clean everything according to the instructions in hot, soapy water. Air-dry the components on a paper towel or a clean dishcloth.

How to Store Your Milk

If you choose to start expressing your milk early or you are trying to build up your supply, it is important to know how to store it. If your milk is not immediately given to your baby, it can be stored at room temperature, refrigerated, or frozen. Each storage procedure requires different handling. Temperature is the single most important factor in determining the length of time it's safe to store your milk.

Storage Time Guidelines

Room Temperature	6–10 hours
Refrigerator	5–8 days
Freezer Inside a Refrigerator	2 weeks
Self-Defrosting Freezer w/Separate Door	3–6 months
Deep Freeze at 0 degrees	6–12 months

Defrosted or thawed milk can be stored for up to twenty-four hours in the refrigerator. If you don't have a refrigerator at your work site, you can refrigerate milk in an insulated cooler with ice packs until you get home or to the daycare.

Store your cooled or frozen milk in the back of your refrigerator. It's cooler there and your milk will be less affected by temperature changes from the frequent opening and closing of the door.

Magical breastmilk does it again! Studies have found that the antibacterial properties of breastmilk actually protect it from bacterial growth while it's stored in a bottle. That's why human milk can be stored at room temperature for up to ten hours. However, if you don't intend to use your milk for some time, it's best refrigerated. Discard any unused portion left in the bottle after your baby has eaten. It's hard to watch that liquid gold go down the drain, but bacteria from your baby's mouth make it unsafe for future feedings.

Plastic versus Glass Debate

For years, people have been debating whether to use plastic or glass bottles. Every couple of years

Mommy Must

If your infant is premature or critically ill, she will require different breastmilk handling and storage techniques than a full-term, healthy infant. You can consult your hospital lactation consultant or NICU staff member to help you express and store your milk properly.

breastfeeding educators learn about new studies that change the recommended practice for storing human milk. Today, new plastics have been developed in response to chemical leakage concerns and using plastic is now considered the best practice.

Plastic—If you're freezing breastmilk in plastic bottles or liner bags, leave at least an inch at the top. As liquids freeze, they expand. Mark the date and amount on the outside of the bottle or bag. You can use wax pencils or masking tape. Be sure to add your baby's name if the bottle will be used at a daycare center. If you're freezing breastmilk in a bottle liner, double bag your milk to decrease the chances of seam leakage. If you have an extra bottle handy, freeze milk with bags still in the bottle to preserve their shape. Bottle liners that are intended for the long-term storage of human milk are the best.

Freeze milk in amounts of two to four ounces. That way, it will thaw more quickly and less will go to waste. When baby consistently takes eight ounces at a single feeding, you can safely freeze your milk in larger amounts, but larger amounts take longer to thaw.

Glass—Glass bottles have long been the storage container of choice for lactation consultants and breastfeeding educators. Because milk expands when frozen, be careful to leave adequate space available in the bottle for this process. Glass bottles can break if you fill them all the way to the top. Again, freeze in smaller amounts.

Ice Cube Trays—Metal ice cube trays can be purchased at gourmet food stores. Simply pour liquid into the tray and seal the whole thing inside a large freezer bag, or cover it tightly with plastic wrap or aluminum foil. Pop out the cubes as needed. If the cubes are too large to fit into the mouth of the bottle, thaw them inside the refrigerator in another container and transfer the milk to a bottle when it's ready.

Containers should be clean, but they don't need to be sterilized. If you have a sick or hospitalized infant, talk to a lactation consultant or NICU personnel. Wash containers and all pumping equipment in hot, soapy water and let them air dry on a paper towel or clean dishcloth. You don't need to wash tubes or other components of the breast pump if they haven't come in contact with your milk.

How to Thaw Frozen Breastmilk

The recommendation for thawing breastmilk is to let it stand in the refrigerator overnight. Milk will thaw slowly and consistently over a twelve-hour period, and faster if frozen in smaller amounts.

Another common method of thawing milk is to place a bottle of frozen milk in a pan of warm water and change the water frequently to replace any lost heat.

Heating Fresh Milk

Your breastmilk is the perfect temperature for your baby. Even when it's been stored at room temperature, fresh milk doesn't need to be heated. Boiling causes it to lose its precious immunity-enhancing properties. Even a slight warm-up in the microwave can hurt the milk and possibly harm your baby. Microwave heat is uneven and causes hot spots in a bottle that will scald baby's mouth. If you decide to refrigerate your milk, you can heat it by holding the bottle under warm tap water or letting it stand in a bowl or pan of warm water.

Supplies and Keeping Them Clean

If you've been nursing your baby at all, way to go! You've given your baby a loving, healthy start. If you're going to bottle-feed now, you need to make a few informed decisions. Are you going to continue with breastmilk or switch to formula, or use both? If you choose to add formula to your routine, how does that work? And then there are bottles and nipples to consider.

Mindful Mommy
This is not the time to be frugal. If your baby finishes her meal and some milk is left, you can't save it for later. Don't refreeze thawed milk or reheat heated milk. To ensure your baby's safety, throw away any milk remaining in her bottle and always use the oldest milk first.

Whether you are incorporating formula into your routine, or need bottles for expressed milk, your considerations will be the same: comfort and safety for your child, and simplicity for you. Remember that your child is used to your breast, so it's important to find a product that he can adjust to easily.

Picking the Right Bottle

Whether you choose to use plastic or glass bottles is up to you. Glass is the preferred material for breast-milk, but either is fine for formula. Bottles come in two basic styles: liner bottles and traditional.

Liner bottles use disposable sterile bags. The liner fits on the inside of a bottomless tube "bottle." Once you screw the nipple on the top and squeeze any extra air out of the bottle liner, you have a bottle baby can drink from in any position. Your baby is also less likely to suck air, thus preventing spitting up or tummy aches.

Nipple Choice

The single most important thing to consider when choosing a nipple is the flow speed. A nipple

Mommy Knows Best

Babies that have been breastfed exclusively for at least twelve months don't need a bottle and should be ready to go straight to a cup or straw. If you introduced the cup at six months, she's probably an old pro by now. It's easier to wean a baby just once!

that lets too much formula out too fast can choke your newborn or let her take in too much air. A low-flow nipple is perfect for newborns. However, your older child may grow frustrated if she has to work too hard at sucking. Check packaging labels for the flow rate when purchasing new nipples.

Once you've selected the proper flow rate for your baby, it's time to let your baby make some choices. In our experience, every baby has a preference for one type of bottle nipple over the others. When you find what she likes, stick with it.

Having said that, here's a quick look at the different nipples available.

Wide-based—Most Playtex liner-style bottles use either a rounded or squared-off, wide-based, soft nipple. If you thought breastfed babies sucked only on Mom's nipples, you'd probably think Playtex was the most naturally shaped bottle nipple. It's not. However, if you're exclusively bottle feeding, that's no big deal. If you prefer a more natural shape but like the Playtex disposable bottle system, you're in luck. Playtex makes orthodontic nipples, too.

Mommy Must

Bottle nipples can wear out. In order to check, take a look at the flow rate of bottle nipples regularly. Fill the bottle, hold it upside down, and observe. The nipple should drip one drop per second. If the liquid streams, the nipple is probably worn out. If you need to squeeze the nipple before it drips, it might be clogged.

Orthodontic—Orthodontic nipples are shaped to resemble what a mother's nipple and areola look like inside a nursing baby's mouth. They are longer and flatter than standard bottle nipples. They come in two sizes. Number 1 is small and designed for premature infants and smaller newborns. Number 2 is fine for most other babies. Orthodontic nipples are called orthodontic because they might help your child's mouth and jaw grow more naturally, as if she were breastfed. Bear in mind that the whole nipple goes into the baby's mouth, not just the tip. There is also a top and bottom to some orthodontic nipples. If you put them into baby's mouth upside down, not much formula can get out. Although orthodontic nipples might be more like real breastfeeding, some babies gag and refuse to use them.

Standard—Standard bottle nipples are inexpensive, easy to find, and can work as well as any other style when properly used. Lately, there's been an explosion in variety of these "old-fashioned" nipples. You can buy them made from a variety of materials, angled or with air-excluding valve systems.

For many years, bottle nipples were manufactured from rubber. Today, silicone has become the material of choice for many parents. Silicone lasts longer than rubber or latex. Unlike traditional materials, silicone has no taste or odor. It's also transparent, so you can see how much milk is in the nipple and be confident that the nipple is clean.

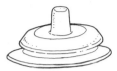

Wide-Based: This style nipple usually works best for babies who have never breastfed.

Orthodontic: Orthodontic nipples are designed to most closely resemble the shape a mother's areola and nipple take in a nursing infant's mouth.

Standard: Standard-shaped nipples are the most basic design and can be as effective as any other style.

Make it a habit to check nipples for wear and deterioration at every cleaning. Grasp the nipple between your thumb and forefinger. Hold the base with your other hand and pull. The nipple should snap back firmly. Immediately replace any torn, sticky, swollen, or cracked bottle nipples.

Keeping Everything Clean

Bottles and nipples should be as clean as possible. And the best way to clean what your baby puts in her mouth is by using boiled water. If you normally wash dishes with unchlorinated water, or if your baby is a preemie, or has weakened immunity, everything needs to be boiled. Bring a pan of water to a full, rolling boil and drop in nipples, bottles, and other utensils that come in contact with your child's food. Let these items boil for five minutes. After everything's cooled, wash your hands well with soap and prepare the bottles.

If you live in a city with chlorinated water, you need to boil only new nipples, once, to remove any chemicals left over from the manufacturing process. After the first use, you can wash them in the sink or top rack of the dishwasher.

Water

It's important to remember that the formula you choose is only part of what your baby will be consuming. The other part is water. Safe water is vital for babies using formula.

How can you be sure your water is safe enough? As a rule, if your city's water supply meets federal and state guidelines for safety, it should be fine for use in formula preparation. However, there are exceptions, so have your water tested if you live in rural areas or have had seasonal thaws or floods.

Mommy Must

You should make a habit of wiping the top of the formula can with a clean cloth before opening it. As with any canned food, you can be confident that the contents of the can are sanitary, but you don't know what's been on the outside.

Many new parents choose bottled water for their babies' formula, but don't be fooled into assuming it's better than the water coming out of your tap at home. The federal regulations for bottled water are far less stringent than the regulations for your city's tap water. A water filter is another option. A simple pitcher purifier can be purchased cheaply and can hold enough water for a day's worth of formula.

Formula Facts

Because there are many different types and brands of infant formula, it's a good idea to talk to your doctor before you feed your little one anything besides breastmilk. Although all types of formula have to be approved by the FDA as safe and nutritious for babies, there are differences to consider based on your baby's individual needs.

Cows'-Milk-Based Formula

This is the meat and potatoes of formulas. It's standard fare for most formula-fed babies from birth to their first birthday. Vitamins, minerals, fats, and

Mommy Knows Best

These days, everyone is buying bottled water. But that gets expensive! Because water can contain lead, minerals, and bacteria, make sure to take precautions before giving it to your child. There are lots of purifiers on the market today, so you'll have a lot to choose from.

sugars are mixed together in a base of cows' milk proteins. If your baby is normal birthweight and healthy, and if you have no reason to suspect food allergies, a regular formula based on modified cows' milk is usually the right choice.

Soy-Based Formula

If your baby is extremely fussy, gassy, or spits up often, talk to your doctor about the possibility of food allergies or a sensitivity to cows' milk protein. If your doctor thinks cows' milk sensitivity is the problem, she'll probably tell you to switch to a soy-based formula. If you're a vegetarian or need to keep kosher, a soy-based formula is the next best thing to breastmilk.

Preemie Formula

Premature babies need formula with a few extras—extra calories, extra proteins, and extra vitamins and minerals. Preemie formulas provide these extras while building on a foundation of milk-based formula. Use of a preemie formula typically begins in the hospital and continues until your doctor recommends a change. Often, babies will be switched to a regular formula once they have caught up with other babies their age in terms of size, weight, and energy.

Predigested Formula

The proteins in predigested formula have been broken down so baby can more easily use them. These formulas are useful for colicky babies or others who might have a sensitivity to milk proteins. Although milk-based, these formulas are specially modified to meet the nutritional needs of special babies. Enfamil Pregestimil goes an extra step and provides 55 percent of its fat content in an easier-to-digest form, too. All the predigested formulas are easier on baby's tummy than regular formula. Baby's less fussy, so Mom and Dad are happier, and the formula company's happier because this stuff costs a mint.

Low-Iron Formula

Low-iron formula has less than the recommended daily allowance of iron for your baby. The AAP does not recommend low-iron formula for infants younger than six months of age. Once upon a time, iron was thought to cause constipation in infants, but that's no longer the case. Anemia (low levels of iron in the blood) is the real health threat for growing babies. Use iron-fortified formula until your baby is old enough to get iron from other sources.

Thickened Formula

Thickened formula is recommended only as a last resort for special needs infants. Never use it without a doctor's recommendation. The thickening agent is a modified rice starch. Although approved for babies from birth to twelve months, cereal products like rice starch ordinarily have no place in an infant's diet before four to six months of age. Their little digestive systems are just not up to it. Thickened formulas can be difficult to mix and they sometimes cause large, smelly stools. On the other hand, thickened formulas can be a lifesaver to certain special needs babies who have trouble keeping formula down. Babies with uncomplicated GER are the most likely candidates for a thickened formula.

Follow-Up Formulas

After your baby celebrates her first birthday, she's ready to move beyond formula. Along with all of the wonderful new foods your baby's been trying since she was six months old, your baby can now drink milk— plain, ordinary homogenized whole milk. Follow-up formulas are marketed to parents who are worried about their baby's nutrition. Some follow-ups are marketed to parents of children as young as four months. There is really no reason to switch away from a regular formula at such a young age. If your little one is getting proper nutrition in her diet after her first birthday, follow-up formulas are an unnecessary expense.

Bottle-Feeding Facts

Your first step should be to get comfortable. Find a place where you can easily support the baby for a length of time without straining yourself. Second, tilt the bottle so the nipple is full of formula. Otherwise your baby will swallow excessive amounts of air during feeding. More air equals more spitup.

Third, tilt your baby so that her head is higher than her stomach. Never feed your baby when she is lying down. She can get ear infections. The eustachian tubes connect your baby's mouth and inner ear. When she drinks lying back, fluids run into her inner ear and stay there. Any food warmed to body temperature is like a fertility clinic for bacteria. Sitting up or reclining slightly are the correct positions for feeding.

Fourth, cuddle your baby. Hold her as if you were breastfeeding. This is especially true for newborns. A newborn's eyes can't focus well beyond about a foot or so. That just happens to be the distance between your eyes and hers when she is breastfeeding. Your baby wants to see you. She wants to interact with you and get to know you. Cuddle your baby while she eats. Coo to her. Sing to her. Take off your shirt and go skin to skin.

These activities bring security and comfort to your baby and help you to bond. Sometimes it might seem like you've been feeding her forever, but you'll look back on those early feedings fondly when your little baby isn't so little anymore.

As your baby becomes able to grasp the bottle and take control, let her. Her coordination might be lacking at first. Sometimes babies frustrate themselves by knocking the bottle out of their own mouths. At those times, hold the bottle but let her grasp and tug it around. Before long, she'll be an old pro

Mommy Knows Best

Even if your baby only has one small tooth, it's time to begin practicing a good dental routine. Make a game of cleaning that precious little tooth. Buy a soft, child-sized toothbrush or use a wet cloth. You don't need toothpaste at this age. Remember, the goal is to take care of the teeth while getting your child into the habit of good dental hygiene.

Chapter 9

What Should I Eat?

FOR MONTHS YOU HAVE been eating for two and now that you are breastfeeding, it's not that different! Breastfeeding moms have nutritional needs above and beyond those of other women. Your milk quality won't usually suffer from poor eating habits, but your own health might. So for you own good, eat well! Your body will provide your baby with all the nutrients she needs, even if it means taking them from you. Many women don't eat a well-balanced diet, so their bodies rob themselves of important nutrients in order to supply the growing infants' needs.

Be a Healthy Example

As your child gets older, she will pick up on your eating habits. When she sees you enjoying good food, she's more likely to enjoy it herself. If you don't like a particular vegetable, she'll pick up on that, too. Getting your child started with a healthy lifestyle is the loving thing to do, and it can be as simple as having healthy food around the house instead of chips and candy.

Fathers can help, too. It's hard to maintain healthy eating habits if your mate isn't following the game plan. Dads should try to stick with a healthy menu around their wives and children whenever possible. It's all too easy to let either parent's bad habit become the family's bad habit. An occasional treat is fine, but if you feel the need to indulge in junk food, practice moderation.

Drink Plenty of Water

It is important for you to stay hydrated while you are breastfeeding your little one. During lactation, your body uses tremendous amounts of water. While mild dehydration on your part won't affect your milk production in any significant way, it can cause problems for your own overall health. Irritability and a loss of energy and focus are some common symptoms of dehydration.

Mommy Must

To stay hydrated, water is the recommended beverage. Juice and soft drinks are too sugary and don't replace your body's fluids as well as water does. A glass or two of fruit juice per day is a healthy addition to your diet, but to avoid unwanted weight gain, dilute juice with water.

You'll begin to feel thirsty only moments after sitting down to breastfeed. Almost every woman does. So get in the habit of taking a glass of water with you every time you nurse. When your baby takes the fluid out, you put it right back in.

Don't wait until you're thirsty to have a glass of water. Thirst is a late indicator of dehydration. Usually, by the time you feel thirsty, your body is already too dry. If your urine is consistently dark, your mouth is dry, and you suffer from constipation, you're probably dehydrated. Stay ahead of dehydration by drinking eight to ten glasses of water every day, but don't overdo it. Extra water won't increase your milk production.

The Food Pyramid, a Pathway to Health

The U.S. Food and Drug Administration publishes the Food Guide Pyramid that we all learned about back in elementary school. It's a handy way to put together a healthy daily menu. The pyramid is built from six food groups.

While reviewing nutrition facts on food packaging, be aware that the suggested serving sizes listed reflect the amount of food that the producer considers to be one serving. The serving size recommended by the Food Guide Pyramid is based on the amount of the food necessary for your nutritional needs.

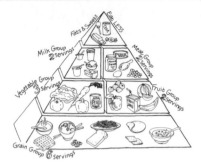

Food Pyramid: The FDA does ongoing research on nutrition and provides the public with tools to ensure its healthy eating habits. Use the Food Pyramid as a guide for yourself, and speak with your pediatrician about a similar guide for your child.

Vitamins and Minerals You Need

It's not always easy to eat a balanced diet but the best way to fulfill all your nutritional requirements is by eating a varied diet from the lower five groups of the Food Pyramid. Whole foods are complex power-houses of good things for your body. A vitamin C pill might provide all of your required vitamin C, but an orange provides the same benefit as a pill along with fiber, carotene, calcium, simple sugars, and more. Many of the components of whole foods might help us in ways that haven't been discovered yet. We just don't know all there is to know about nutrition. Without a complete knowledge of our nutritional needs, we can't presume to fill those needs with an artificial supplement.

Another reason whole foods are superior to supplements is the availability of the nutrients to your body. It's not enough for a pill to contain 100 percent of your daily vitamin and mineral needs if those nutrients are provided in a form your body can't easily use. The availability of nutrients is sometimes strongly affected by the presence of other nutrients. A multivitamin and mineral pill contains ingredients that get in each other's way. For instance, high doses of iron will interfere with your body's ability to absorb zinc and copper.

That's not to say you shouldn't take a daily supplement, but a pill is not a fix for poor eating habits. Think of vitamin and mineral pills as a way to increase your chances of getting all the nutrients you need. Your prenatal supplement is a good source of nutrients that might help to fill in the blanks on your body's nutritional checklist. Avoid taking any additional supplements without the approval of your health care provider.

Mindful Mommy

Too much of a good thing can be harmful! So don't overdo it. For example, excessive vitamin D can cause symptoms ranging from nausea to kidney failure. Too much vitamin A can lead to headaches, hair loss, and liver damage. Watch what you are eating and avoid supplements unless you really need them!

What to Avoid

Although most women can eat anything they want while breastfeeding without any problems, some foods have a bad reputation among nursing mothers. These foods can pass into your breastmilk and change its flavor or cause allergic reactions in your baby. Symptoms vary but usually involve fussiness, an unwillingness to nurse, rash, diarrhea, or vomiting. Often, a baby who suddenly refuses to nurse is responding to the flavor of your milk. If your baby displays any of these symptoms, examine your diet and check it against this list of the usual suspects.

- Caffeine
- Chocolate
- Citrus fruits
- Dairy products
- Foods that cause you gas
- Nuts (especially peanuts)
- Spicy foods

Eliminating these foods from your diet might help. However, the change in your baby will not be immediate. To find the offending food, try cutting out one of the possible culprits from your diet for a week or two. If your baby's symptoms persist, try eliminating the next food.

Once you identify a problem food, keep it off your menu for a few months. Older babies can more easily tolerate a variety of flavors. Another solution is to avoid large amounts of any one food at a time. Some women find they are able to eat small amounts of their problem foods if they don't do it very often. No two women are the same, so you'll have to experiment a little.

Honing In on Healthy Snacks

With a new baby in the house, or any other time, it's not always easy to prepare regular meals. Luckily, good nutrition is just as easy to achieve by "grazing" as it is by eating three square meals every day. Keeping healthy snacks on hand is a great way to get your recommended daily allowances (RDAs), keep off unwanted weight, and set a good lifelong example for your child. Instead of chips or cookies, try some of the following quick and healthy alternatives or add your own from the Food Pyramid.

- Apples
- Bananas
- Breads (tortillas, bagels, biscuits, muffins, breads)
- Cantaloupe
- Carrot sticks
- Celery
- Cereal
- Crackers
- Eggs
- Grapes
- Oranges
- Plums
- Popcorn (plain)
- Salads
- Soups
- Strawberries
- Tomatoes (may cause gas)
- Yogurt

Special Diet Concerns

You may, for a variety of reasons, have a special diet. Whether you're a vegetarian or have medical restrictions, you'll want to take extra care. Special attention is important not only for your baby's nutrition, but also to preserve your own health. If you need additional information, consult your doctor or a nutritionist.

Vegetarian Diet

If you're a vegetarian, you already pay special attention to your diet. You have an advantage because you already know what it's like to watch what you eat and consider all of the components. Your nutritional needs will depend on which type of vegetarian you are.

Lacto-ovo vegetarians, who eat eggs and dairy products, can generally meet all their nutritional needs from food sources. However, vegans, those vegetarians who don't eat any animal products at all, are at risk for nutritional deficiencies in several important areas. Protein, vitamin D, riboflavin, calcium, iron, and zinc are harder to find in plant form than in animal products, but it can be done.

Vitamin B_{12} does not naturally occur in plant sources, and vegans, lactating or not, need to supplement this important nutrient.

There is also some question about the availability of important, brain-nourishing fats like DHA in strict vegan diets. Noted pediatric experts Martha and

William Sears believe so strongly in the importance of DHA in a breastfeeding mom's diet that they recommend vegans temporarily add fish to their daily menu.

Consider the following suggestions of good dietary sources for the nutrients most often lacking in vegetarian diets.

Where to Find Essential Vitamins, Minerals, and Proteins	
Vitamins	
B_{12}	fortified soy beverages and cereals
D	fortified soy beverages and sunshine
Riboflavin (B_2)	fortified whole grains, avocados, and nuts
Minerals	
Calcium	soy beverages, calcium-enriched orange juice, broccoli, nuts, seeds, bok choy, greens, grains, peas and beans, kale, and some tofu
Iron	green leafy vegetables, iron-fortified cereals and breads, peas, beans, tofu, dried fruits, and whole grains
Zinc	tofu, nuts, peas, beans, wheat germ, bran, whole grain breads
Proteins	soy, nuts, seeds, peas, beans, grains, and vegetables

The continued use of a prenatal vitamin and mineral supplement while nursing is an especially good idea for vegetarian mothers.

Teen Moms

If you are a teen mother, you may still be growing yourself. It is important for mothers below the age of nineteen to address their additional nutritional needs. The U.S. Department of Agriculture (USDA) recommends additional calcium, phosphorus, and magnesium for teen moms. Phosphorus works with calcium to form teeth and bones. Magnesium is necessary in the production of healthy bones, teeth, and nerves. Magnesium also helps prevent heart attacks and stroke. Teen mothers should make special efforts to incorporate the following into their diet:

- **Calcium:** Milk, cheese, whole grains, egg yolk, peas, beans, nuts, green leafy vegetables
- **Phosphorus:** Milk, cheese, meat, egg yolk, whole grains, peas, beans, nuts
- **Magnesium:** dark green leafy vegetables, bananas, dried apricots, avocados, cashews, almonds, soy products, whole grains, chocolate

In addition to focusing on the previous elements, very young mothers should be diligent about taking their prenatal vitamins and having regular OB visits.

Weight-Loss Plans You Can Stick To

As a new mother, you are probably looking forward to regaining your original shape, if it's possible! And luckily, breastfeeding is a wonderful, natural weight-loss plan. Studies consistently show that women who nurse their babies return to their pre-pregnancy weight faster than moms who formula-feed. All the fat cells your body stockpiled during pregnancy, and even some from before, will be used to make milk for your baby.

When you breastfeed, your body needs about 500 extra calories every day. That means you can eat a little bit more than usual and still lose weight. If you only consume an extra 300 calories every day, your body will use your fat stores to make up the difference.

Your weight loss while breastfeeding will be slow but steady. That's the way nature intended it. Crash dieting puts you at risk for nutritional deficiencies and might eventually affect the quality of your milk. Besides, crash diets don't work. Studies show that rapid weight loss at any time of life is usually followed by rapid weight gain. The best way to keep weight off is to lose it gradually through a combination of diet and exercise.

Choosing healthy foods and drinking lots of water during lactation will get you into the right habits. Keep your weight loss down to one pound per week or less. Even half a pound per week will melt away those pregnancy pounds within a year.

Mindful Mommy

Before changing your diet, consult a doctor if you have preexisting medical conditions. Especially if you are on a restricted diet of any kind, talk with your health care provider before making any changes. Even a vitamin and mineral pill can cause problems for some people.

Chapter 10

Should I Exercise?

MANY WOMEN WONDER IF exercise is good for them while they are breastfeeding. Well, it is! In general, anything that helps a nursing mother stay confident and ward off depression will also help her have a positive breastfeeding experience. Your mind and body have far-reaching effects on each other, and that connection can make all the difference in the quality of your life. It's vital to realize that exercise is not only compatible with lactation, it's beneficial as well.

The Benefits of Exercise

This might not feel like the best time to start or resume a program of regular exercise, but exercise can help you in every part of your life, including breastfeeding. As little as twenty to thirty minutes of aerobic exercise three or four times per week can help you feel better, look better, and live longer. Performing toning exercises like sit-ups and leg lifts can help your body regain its pre-pregnancy shape more quickly. Any amount of exercise will burn up calories and help you lose some of that leftover pregnancy weight.

Exercise:

- Increases your energy level
- Steps up your metabolism so you burn more calories even at rest
- Tones your muscles
- Gives you a sense of accomplishment that boosts your confidence
- Improves your circulation
- Fights off depression and boredom
- Helps you to lose weight
- Makes you feel sexier
- Sets a good example for your child as he grows

Make sure that you don't get ahead of yourself though. As important as exercise is, it can be dangerous to overdo it! Weight loss should be very gradual in breastfeeding women. One pound per week is the maximum. If you're losing more than that, you're putting yourself and your baby at risk for nutritional deficiencies. Exercise for health, not just weight loss.

Remember to always stretch before and after a workout. Stretching lengthens your muscles, increases your flexibility, and greatly reduces your chance of injury. You'll also find stretching helpful in relieving muscle cramps and other muscle-related pains.

When to Start

How and when to start are questions that you and your doctor should discuss. In fact, before beginning any exercise program, it is important to consult your physician. There are conditions, like Caesarean section delivery and abdominal diastasis that might keep you more sedentary than you would like. Adequate recovery time and sometimes specialized exercise routines are absolute necessities to avoid dangerous complications.

Doctors generally advise women without special conditions to wait at least six weeks after delivery before beginning or resuming an aerobic exercise program. Your body needs the time both to recover from childbearing and to establish a good milk supply. You and your baby also need those first weeks to work out a nursing routine.

However, that doesn't mean you're on bed rest. Shaping and toning exercises are generally all right. Sit-ups and leg lifts can help your body recover. You can also go about any normal activity that doesn't cause you pain or undue stress. Walking is a great all-around exercise anytime. Many women are out of bed and walking the hospital halls an hour after their babies are born. Just take it slow and work your way up to the level of activity you want.

Mommy Knows Best

Many women experience the unpleasantness of diastasis as a result of labor. It occurs when the vertical muscles in your abdomen separate. The condition will heal with time, but be careful because even mild exertion can make it worse. Some health professionals recommend a very gentle exercise that resembles a sit-up without the "up" part. Talk to your doctor to find out.

Take Time for You

With a newborn, it's easy to get so busy that you forget to take care of yourself. With all the new responsibilities of parenthood, clearing your schedule at a certain time every day or two for exercise isn't always practical. Your baby needs to be fed, changed, and held. Your toddler needs attention, stimulation, and socialization. The dog needs to be walked. Everyone else's needs seem to come first. As a result, in those busy first months, you've got to become an exercise opportunist.

Make exercise part of your ordinary activities. Three 10-minute chunks of time are as effective as thirty minutes in a row. Shorter stretches are easier to get through and easier to schedule. Even little activities that seem like they wouldn't make much of a difference add up quickly over the course of a few months.

As you surely know, your body went through some major changes during the last couple of months. Well, now that you are breastfeeding, lactation adds new and different demands. Your body isn't the same

Mommy Knows Best

It's a common myth that if you wake up early to exercise, you will just be more tired! On the contrary, you'll find that you're energized, not exhausted. Give it a shot; try getting up half an hour before your baby's usual wake-up time and work out.

as it was before pregnancy, and you've got to keep that in mind as you exercise.

The American College of Obstetricians and Gynecologists has issued guidelines for exercise during the weeks after childbirth.

1. Exercise regularly, at least three times per week. If you're playing a sport, don't compete.
2. Don't exercise too hard in hot, humid weather or when you have a fever.
3. Keep your movements smooth. Don't bounce or jerk. Exercise on a wooden floor or a tightly carpeted surface.
4. Your joints are looser than normal, so avoid flexing or extending them very far. Loose joints can lead to dislocation or damage, so avoid jumping, jarring, or rapid changes in direction.
5. Always warm up for five minutes before any vigorous workout. Slow walking is a good warm-up.
6. At the end of a workout, slow down gradually and stretch. However, because your joints are looser than normal, don't stretch any joint to its maximum position.
7. Women should monitor their heart rates and stay within the range advised by their doctors.
8. Rise slowly. There's an increased risk of fainting due to sudden changes in your blood pressure. Work your legs gently for a few minutes after you get back on your feet.

9. Drink plenty of water to avoid dehydration. Drink whenever you're thirsty, even if it means interrupting the workout.

10. If you haven't been very active in the past, you should start slowly and increase your workout over time.

11. At the first sign of unusual symptoms, you should stop exercising and contact your doctor.

Lactating moms need to take some other precautions as well. Nurse your baby or express your milk before working out and wear a good, supportive sports bra. Full breasts can be painful if they are jostled around too much.

After a workout, immediately remove your bra. Wash your breasts with plain water and let them air dry. A sweaty breast might be unappealingly salty to your baby, and clean, dry breasts are much less likely to become infected from clogged milk ducts.

How Exercise Affects Breastmilk

Throughout the past couple of years, some people have reported that exercise sours breastmilk and leads to fussy babies that reject the breast. But recent studies show that this is simply not true. All the speculation is based on a single study that compared breastmilk samples taken before and after exhaustive exercise sessions.

In that study, it was observed that babies seemed less eager to take breastmilk immediately after their moms had worked out to near-exhaustion. Researchers blamed lactic acid, a normal by-product of exercise, for the effect. That's as much information as most of the public received. Less known is that the effect lasted for only about one hour. So, if your exercise routine involves pushing on to the point of exhaustion, you might want to wait an hour before feeding your child. Otherwise, you really don't need to worry about any negative effects to your milk.

Exercises to Do with Your Baby

There are various exercises that you can do with your child. In fact, children love to move and play! And they especially love to move and play with their mommies. Involving your baby or toddler in your exercise routine makes working out fun and it's a great way to get closer to your child. Here are some ideas for exercising with your little one:

- Put your baby in a sling or a stroller and go for a long family walk. You can walk through the park, around the mall, or just around your neighborhood.
- Buy a jogging stroller with big bicycle tires and take your child on a run.
- Buy a bike trailer and take him for a ride.
- Pull your toddler behind you in a wagon.

- Do sit-ups in front of your baby in a bouncy swing, and say "peek-a-boo" every time you come forward. He'll love it!
- Lie on the floor next to your baby and do leg lifts. It's a great way to exercise while still maintaining face-to-face contact.
- Dance with your child in your arms—slow or fast or anywhere in between.
- Use your baby as a weight. When she is old enough to support her head, lift her up while you're lying on the floor. Bring her to your nose with a smile and some words of love, then put her back out at arm's length and do it again.

Toddlers can be a workout all by themselves. Just try to keep up with yours for a while! If you really want a workout, take your toddler to the home of a friend who doesn't have children. People without kids always have lots of breakable things within a toddler's easy reach. By the time you've followed two steps behind your curious youngster for an hour, you'll feel like you've run a marathon.

Sex and the Breastfeeding Couple

While you are breastfeeding your baby, it is normal to think about the meaning and importance of breasts. While American culture loves to emphasize the sexuality of the breasts, some people, even health care professionals, want to desexualize the breast entirely.

They point out that breasts are clearly designed to feed babies and that's serious business. Your breasts are wonderful sources of nourishment and emotional comfort for your baby, but they're sexual, too. Your challenge is to find the balance that works for you and your partner.

People who want to desexualize breasts are usually reacting to the way sexuality can interfere with breastfeeding. For instance, some husbands find it difficult at first to share their partner's breasts with a baby. They might be unwilling to accommodate any other use for their private playground. It seems like everything from public nursing to our most private thoughts and feelings about breastfeeding can get all tangled up in our attitudes about sex.

Let's state right here that, yes, breasts are sexual—but your whole body is sexual. When it comes to making a body part sexual, it's in the way that you use it. In many cultures, breasts are just one more piece of a woman's anatomy, like an arm or a leg. There are cultures (and individuals) that find a well-turned ankle, the eyes, or even a quick mind far more exciting than an exposed breast.

Mommy Knows Best

You're not a bad mother if you occasionally become sexually aroused while breastfeeding. It's normal! Oxytocin, the hormone released by your body when baby suckles, is also released during sex. Some women even reach orgasm. Breastfeeding is a pleasurable experience. It's one of nature's rewards.

Speaking of minds, the brain is your most important sexual organ. Sex is a combination of friction and fantasy. For some men, part of the thrill of breasts is the context in which they have access to them. If your husband is one of these guys, he might only be used to seeing your breasts during sexual encounters.

So, now are your breasts only for the baby? No, not if you're comfortable with breast play as a part of your sexual relationship with your mate. Your breasts can be less sensitive, overly sensitive, or unchanged in the weeks following birth. All of these conditions are normal. If you enjoy the contact, there's no reason you can't resume breast play.

Sex: Let's Talk About It

There are many things to consider before having sex for the first time after labor. You might want to consult your doctor or midwife to talk about your progress and recovery before you do anything. Generally speaking though, most American doctors advise new parents to wait at least six weeks after birth before having sex. In other countries, a three-week wait is standard. In any case, your body needs some time to heal. The placental separation from the uterine wall

Mommy Must

Many women don't want to think about sex immediately following the birth of their baby. The lack of interest is often due to hormonal changes that serve to focus a new mother's attention on the baby. It's a temporary condition, but combined with sleep deprivation, it can leave little room for romance.

must heal. Tears or episiotomy incisions take time to repair and become flexible again. Six weeks might not be enough time for all of that to happen.

When It's Time

Eventually, you'll feel ready for intercourse and when you do, you'll need to take a few special precautions. That first time after childbirth is a lot like your other first time. The experience can be anywhere from mildly uncomfortable to downright painful. To lessen the stress and pain, try the following:

- Relax. In her popular book, *The Girlfriends' Guide to Surviving the First Year of Motherhood*, Vicki McCarty Lovine recommends that you "inebriate and lubricate." That advice might work for some women, but breastfeeding mothers need to be careful about using a glass of wine or any other alcoholic beverage to help them relax. Refer to Chapter Two to read about breastfeeding and drinking.
- Pay attention to lubrication. Postpartum estrogen levels reduce your vagina's natural lubrication, so have a tube of the artificial stuff

Mommy Knows Best

Numbers and norms vary among women, but it is interesting to note that research has clearly shown that breastfeeding speeds recovery from pregnancy and childbirth. A faster recovery would seem to naturally favor a more immediate return to sexual readiness.

on hand. K-Y jelly and Astroglide are good choices. Spermicidal jellies are another. Normal amounts of lubrication usually return after your first menstrual cycle.

- Use birth control. You might need to try a different method than usual while breastfeeding. Consult the sections on birth control that follow for advice.

- Take the lead. Women generally prefer to be on top or lie side-by-side with their husband (the spoon position) during intercourse. These positions let you control the amount of pressure put on delicate perineal tissue.

- Communicate. Moms, let your husband know what you enjoy and what's just too uncomfortable right now. Don't suffer through the event. Your partner wants you to enjoy yourself.

- Expect some milk leakage. Sexual stimulation releases oxytocin, the hormone that causes your milk ejection, or letdown reflex. Your breasts might leak when you make love and even spray your partner in the face when you orgasm. If that's a problem (and who says it has to be?), nurse your baby before you have sex or wear a bra and nursing pads. In any case, you'll want to keep a towel handy. Those things are loaded and they might just go off!

- Take your time. It's been a while, but a new mom's body is too sensitive to rush things. Dad, you've waited this long, a few more minutes won't hurt. Foreplay should be long and relaxed.

Your Body and Its Changes Since Birthing

After labor, you may feel as if your body is something totally foreign. But don't worry, you will regain a sense of normalcy soon! The weeks and months following the birth of your baby are a time of transition for your body. Internally, your uterus, cervix, and vagina are recovering. Breastfeeding helps. When your baby nurses, you will feel your uterus contract. At first, it can hurt, but after the uterus regains its normal size, those contractions often become pleasurable.

Like your uterus, your vagina was stretched by childbirth. Many women worry that their vaginas will never regain their pre-delivery size and wonder if their husbands will find sex less satisfying than before. However, the vagina is a truly remarkable organ. It can expand to accommodate a baby's head and then shrink back to its normal size in just a few days. If you want to accelerate the process along or just tighten your pelvic muscles. Kegel exercises are very effective.

Mommy Knows Best

Kegel exercises are a great way to firm up the muscles in the pelvic floor. Do them as often as you can. To make sure you're doing it right, occasionally practice while you're urinating.

1. Tense up your vaginal and anal muscles as if you were trying to stop a stream of urine.
2. Hold the tension for five seconds.
3. Relax and repeat three to five times.

Remind the men in your life, there's only one right answer to the question "How do I look?" That answer is "Beautiful." Disparaging comments about your mate's body, even in jest, can destroy the intimacy your relationship needs to pass the test of time. A mother's body isn't the body of a girl. It's a woman's body. It's fuller, softer, and more sensuous.

Breastfeeding and Birth Control

You may be happy to hear that breastfeeding can be considered nature's own form of birth control. If you exclusively breastfeed your baby, you might find that no other contraceptive is necessary. A drop in estrogen production is one of the hormonal changes necessary for milk production to begin and that results in reduced fertility. Doctors call it lactational amenorrhea. Your menstrual cycle stops. Your fertility is so drastically cut that it's like you're using the pill. For a woman with lactational amenorrhea, there's less than a 2 percent chance of conception.

Despite this remarkable contraceptive power, most authorities advise women to use an additional form of birth control to be safe. The reason behind this recommendation is simple. Lactational amenorrhea is easily interrupted, and you might ovulate before the return of your menses. Some women are simply caught off guard.

With precautions, lactational amenorrhea can last at least six months. Some mothers maintain it for much longer. If you plan to rely on breastfeeding as your contraception, here are some guidelines.

- Breastfeed exclusively. Do not supplement with any formula or food, or even a bottle of human milk, for at least the first six months.
- Don't use pacifiers or bottles. Pacify your baby at your breast only.
- Stay as close to your baby as possible. Every woman is different. Some women will begin ovulating again if they are separated from their child for as little as three or four hours. Consider sleeping with your baby or at least close by in the same room.
- Nurse your older baby often. Your baby should breastfeed at least eight times in a twenty-four-hour period. Feed at least every six hours, and keep your total daily suckling time to a minimum of sixty minutes.

When your menses returns or your baby reaches six months of age, the reliability of this natural contraceptive is reduced and you should immediately begin using another form of birth control.

Birth Control Options

If you decide to use contraceptives, you should be aware of the impact that certain methods might have on your breastfeeding experience and, possibly, your baby. The safest choice while nursing is a method that doesn't involve chemicals. That means natural family planning, condoms, diaphragms, and cervical caps and the Copper T IUD. The next best choices are products using spermacides like foams, gels, and sponges.

Avoid contraceptive pills that are high in estrogen. They can reduce your milk production. The more common progestin-only pills are considered safe for breastfeeding mothers, as are progestin injections or subdermal implants. For breastfeeding women, injections like Depo-Provera are slightly less effective than implants like Norplant. Although hormonal steroids have not been shown to pose any risk to your baby, they do pass into your milk in small amounts. Some health care professionals worry about early exposure of infants to these compounds and advise breastfeeding mothers to delay their use.

Talk to your doctor for more information about birth control options.

Chapter 11

How Long Should I Breastfeed?

EVENTUALLY EVERY MOTHER ASKS the same question: "How long should I breastfeed?" Many women find it helpful to talk with their friends, colleagues, and doctors about this but in the end, the decision is yours and yours only! Everyone seems to have an opinion on this one, and most will share it freely. Some folks will warn you against "coddling" older infants and toddlers. Others might think it's "inappropriate" to nurse a child beyond a particular age.

Understanding Your Physical Limits

Physically, women should be able to nurse their children as long as they need to. If milk is being taken from the breast, more milk will be produced to take its place. From puberty to death you can produce milk. Yes, that long!

There's also no physical limit on the age of your nursing child. Although breastmilk is all your baby needs for the first six months of life, older children continue to get immunities and vitamins from your milk for as long as you let them nurse.

Now, just because you can nurse forever doesn't mean you will. Even if you don't actively stop your child from breastfeeding, she will probably stop on her own. If left to the child, breastfeeding usually comes to a natural conclusion by the time they reach three to four years of age. Of course, you can stop long before then if you decide you want to.

What Doctors Recommend

After learning that most women can breastfeed throughout their lives, we are forced to ask the other important question: "How long should I breastfeed?" There are quite a few recommendations from the medical community and, luckily, they all agree.

- The AAP suggests that all babies should breast-feed exclusively for their first six months, and as long after that as the family chooses.
- The ILCA believes that all mothers should nurse exclusively for a minimum of six months, then add other foods and continue to nurse until two years or as long as they can.
- The U.N.'s WHO endorses breastfeeding with no other foods for at least the child's first six months of life. In an April 2001 Note to the Press, however, The WHO ". . . recognizes

that some mothers will be unable to, or choose not to, follow this recommendation."

In short, the medical community says you should breastfeed exclusively for at least your baby's first six months of life. Doctors and researchers recognize the value of breastfeeding with no other supplemental foods for the baby during that first half-year. They also recognize the benefits of continued breastfeeding along with other foods until your baby's second birthday and beyond.

So the simple answer is this: You should nurse your baby for at least the first six months, and continue for as long afterward as both you and your baby want.

What Others Will Think

It is natural to wonder about how other people, perhaps your friends, colleagues, and extended family members, will react to your breastfeeding practice. It is difficult to predict how or why people act the way they do. Throughout the years, the norms have changed in our society.

Today, we're lucky. The pendulum of public opinion has swung back in favor of breastfeeding. Accompanying practices like public nursing, which Americans once considered "primitive" or "unladylike," are becoming increasingly accepted, even unremarkable. At the same time, the increase in popularity that breastfeeding has enjoyed over the past twenty-five years has raised a new generation that's more supportive of lactation.

Despite the many benefits of extending breast-feeding beyond a year, American popular culture seems resistant to the idea. There have even been charges brought against women for nursing school-aged children. No convictions have resulted, but an irrational discomfort with extended nursing is apparent.

Critics of extended breastfeeding believe that it fosters dependence and immaturity. However, growth is a process that can't be rushed. Stability, love, and security are the foundations of healthy growth. Breastfeeding helps a mother nurture her child's development.

Nursing Your Toddler

The benefits of breastfeeding a toddler are no different than they are for younger children. There are many reasons why mothers choose to nurse their toddlers, some of them are as follows:

Mindful Mommy

Some people will criticize your decision to breastfeed beyond your baby's first few months. But it's not their decision! If you feel like getting into it, tell the critic your doctor's recommendations. You might even explain the benefits of nursing. To people who say, "You're still nursing that child?" just smile and tell them, "Yes. And thanks for noticing!"

- Breastmilk continues to be a wonderful source of nutrition, regardless of anything else your child eats.
- Antibodies in your milk continue to protect your toddler, even if he nurses just once a day.
- Breastfeeding comforts children.
- Toddler nursing might be the only snuggle time you get with your busy child while he's awake.
- Breastmilk can be tolerated by sick children who are unable to stomach other foods.

The more you meet your child's needs, the more independent and confident she will grow. Knowing that you're there for her as she continues to explore gives her the courage to take on a huge, exciting unknown world. Every successful mission will bolster her confidence and increase her sense of independence. Breastfeeding helps.

Styles and Tips

If you decide to continue nursing your toddler child, you might face some unique challenges, but they're usually no problem if you know in advance how to deal with them.

First, how will your child let you know when he wants to nurse? A one-year-old who announces that he wants "boobies" might be cute around the house, but when he says the same thing in public it can leave you glowing red with embarrassment. This is a problem you can prevent by choosing a good code word for breastfeeding early in your relationship. "Nurse" is a good one, but anything you like will work.

If you master the name change, your next hurdle will be explaining that you won't be feeding in public so much anymore. With such a general misunderstanding of toddler nursing in America, public feedings can leave you feeling humiliated by the stares and whispers of uninformed strangers. Your child is probably used to nursing whenever he wants. Any new restrictions are bound to evoke a tantrum in a headstrong toddler, so be ready for it. This is a good time to begin explaining the difference between "public" and "private." Or you might choose to confidently nurse in public knowing that you are doing the best for your child.

Nursing Through Your Next Pregnancy

If you are still breastfeeding and you become pregnant, you don't necessarily have to wean. Pregnancy and lactation are more compatible than once

Mommy Knows Best

While your child is at your breast, you should make sure that his hands don't roam. Hold your child's hand and kiss his little fingers or keep a special toy or book nearby that he can hold. A textured rattle is sometimes a good choice. The name of the game is distraction.

believed, and continued breastfeeding helps an older child feel secure during this time of change.

Obstetricians once routinely advised pregnant women to discontinue breastfeeding for fear of a miscarriage. Nipple stimulation caused by suckling releases oxytocin in your body. This hormone causes a number of things to occur, including milk ejection (letdown) and uterine contractions.

Although oxytocin is released in a pregnant mother's body when she nurses her child, the uterine tissues are less receptive to its effects than they would be if she weren't lactating. Current research seems to indicate that this decreased sensitivity to oxytocin stays strong throughout the first four months of pregnancy. Even after that time, you can continue to nurse your older child with confidence as long as everything else about your pregnancy is normal.

Throughout your pregnancy, you and your toddler will have to accommodate some changes. Beginning in about the fourth month, your breastmilk will decrease in volume and begin to change into the colostrum your newborn needs. Your toddler might or might not give any notice to these changes. Some little ones continue right along, nursing like normal.

Mommy Knows Best

There are circumstances in which you should not breastfeed if you are pregnant. For example if you have a history of miscarriages, are diagnosed as "at risk" for early labor, or notice strong contractions while breastfeeding during your pregnancy, you should stop nursing your child.

Others will decide that your milk tastes funny and they'll nurse less frequently.

If you decide to stop breastfeeding, even for a day, it's important for you to find other ways to bond with your toddler. This is also a great opportunity for Dad to spend a little more time with his child. Both parents can read, snuggle, and play more with their toddler whenever breastfeeding is interrupted. These other activities will keep him happy and secure in the knowledge that he's not being replaced. With all of the attention the new baby gets, it's common for your older child to feel left out.

Tandem Nursing—You're Brave!

Tandem nursing is when you breastfeed two or more children at the same time. It's a great way to keep older children connected with Mom and teach the value of sharing.

The term *tandem nursing* is really a misnomer. Most mothers who breastfeed both a newborn and an older child don't do it simultaneously. Usually, the newborn nurses first, and then Mom is available

Mommy Must

During the first few days of your newborn's life, you should let him nurse first and nurse as often as he wants. This system of feeding is important to ensure that he receives all the colostrum he needs.

to breastfeed the older child. While common, this approach is not without its drawbacks.

Like serial nursing of twins and triplets, a mother who feeds her toddler after her newborn might feel like all she does is breastfeed. That can make the process feel less like bonding, and more like an assembly line. Even if you don't mind the arrangement, your toddler might. Depending on how you handled his feedings through your latest pregnancy, your toddler might feel suddenly displaced.

For some moms, simultaneous breastfeeding is the solution. With a child on each breast, nursing takes a lot less time. There's no perceived favorite and both children stay close to Mom. They might even bond with each other more effectively as they share the satisfaction of nursing. If you find that you don't like it, then try something else. There is no right or wrong answer here. The goal is to find a way to keep all of you happy. Ideally, tandem nursing should be a win-win-win situation.

Chapter 12

When Should I Wean?

EVERY BREASTFEEDING MOTHER WILL ask the question. Some wean at six months and others wait until their babies initiate the process. Without a doubt, when to wean depends on both you and your baby. Some babies lose interest in nursing once solids are offered or the cup is introduced. Others nurse happily until they become mobile and begin to move toward independence. Still others are content to nurse throughout their preschool years. The methods you use will differ depending on who's initiating the process.

Whose Decision Is It?

Even if you are on board to keep nursing, some babies, completely out of the blue, decide that they don't want to anymore. He'll purse his lips, refuse the breast, and cry. This might last for one feeding or for several days. It can be hard to tell if your baby is ill, self-weaning, or holding a nursing strike.

The solution? If at first you don't succeed, try, try again. Offer the breast when your baby is sleepy. He is less prone to fight it when he's tired. Offer to nurse again as your baby wakes. The quiet-alert state is best. Some suggest that simply changing feeding positions or nursing while walking helps.

If your baby still refuses to nurse, express your milk and offer it in an infant feeding cup, a spoon, a syringe, an eyedropper, or a sippy cup.

Your milk supply is regulated by your baby's demand. When your baby refuses to nurse, your body slows production. Nursing strikes usually don't exceed four days, but by that time, your milk supply could decrease. To maintain your supply, express milk manually or with a breast pump as often as your baby would normally nurse.

After twenty-four hours of baby's refusal of the breast, it's time to call your doctor or lactation consultant. Your baby might need a checkup to factor out health conditions like thrush or ear infection.

Sudden Weaning

Sometimes your baby will stop breastfeeding suddenly. This kind of abrupt weaning can be difficult and uncomfortable for both mother and baby. It can lead to engorgement and breast infections, as well as feelings of depression and loss for Mom. It can also lead to nipple confusion if your baby is transitioned to a bottle for the first time.

Teething Can Hurt Both of You

The teething process can disrupt the breastfeeding relationship if it's simply too painful for your baby to nurse. Your baby might refuse the breast or she might bite you to help work her teeth through. The initial shock and pain might cause you to reflexively shout, which will, in turn, scare your baby and might cause her to refuse the breast the next time it's offered.

If you're aware of the signs of teething, you can be on guard against biting before it happens. Signs of teething include:

- Biting everything in sight from spoons and sippy cup lids to you and unsuspecting playmates
- Diaper rash from diahrrea caused by the acids in excess saliva.
- Drooling
- Rash or chapped chin
- Tearfulness

Teething does not have to be a reason to wean, although many parents use this event as a time to transition babies to the bottle.

The Emotional Rollercoaster

When a woman stops breastfeeding, it is common for her to feel the baby blues. You might have put off this postpartum phenomenon because you made the decision to breastfeed. But with sudden weaning you may begin to experience these symptoms for the first time. As prolactin levels decrease, you may begin to experience feelings of sadness, teariness, decrease in appetite, confusion, insomnia, and mood swings.

These feelings will pass as your hormones balance out, but it's important to eat right, exercise, take time for yourself, and find a supportive person to talk to.

Stopping Your Milk Production

Stopping breastfeeding cold turkey is usually an unnecessary and often times painful process. Ideally, weaning is a gradual process.

The most likely result of sudden weaning is engorgement. It happens because rapid weaning can leave you with full, painful breasts. When this happens, express just enough milk to make yourself comfortable, but remember that milk is made by supply and demand. When you express milk, it will be replaced with more. Milk remaining in the breast signals your body that you have more milk than you're using, and will slow production.

Mindful Mommy

Pay attention to your health. Because sudden weaning can cause clogged ducts or breast infection, see your doctor or midwife if you experience fever, chills, heat in your breast, or flulike symptoms. You may need to be treated with an antibiotic.

Cabbage Leaves Save the Day, Again

Earlier, you learned that cool cabbage leaves tucked into your bra can relieve engorgement. You also learned not to use them too long or too often because they slow milk production. Now your goal *is* to slow production, so feel free to use them as much as you need to.

Leaves should be changed when they begin to wilt. During weaning, cabbage leaves can be worn around the clock.

Estrogen Effects

Estrogen, as discussed earlier, is a hormone that reduces milk production. Some birth control pills contain high levels of estrogen, which will decrease your milk supply. However, many birth control pills on the market today are estrogen-free. Talk to your doctor before asking for a prescription. Estrogen has been associated with breast cancer, as well as uterine and cervical cancers, so making a decision to take these for weaning may be difficult.

Gradual Weaning

Gradual weaning is the natural process of ending breastfeeding. The first step to gradual weaning is to develop a plan. Look at a calendar to put this in perspective. You'll need six to eight weeks for a comfortable transition. The more time you take, the less traumatic it will be for both you and your child.

Gradual weaning will help you maintain a healthy hormonal balance. Because your hormone levels will decrease more slowly over time, you'll feel fewer symptoms of the baby blues. The key to keeping mood swings in check is proceeding slowly.

A gradual transition will also keep lactation in balance. Mothers who wean slowly don't experience engorgement. Your weaning infant or toddler will help your body produce just the right amount of milk.

Start to Reduce Feedings

When is your baby least interested in nursing? Midmorning? Early evening? Those will be the first feedings to eliminate, but only one at a time. If you decide to wean in two months, plot out sessions to eliminate, as well as new activities or foods to substitute.

Decrease your nursing schedule by one session every five days. For example, eliminate midmorning nursing, and after five days, begin to eliminate early evening sessions. Bedtimes and naptimes will be the last to go because babies often suck for comfort on these occasions. Nighttime feedings are

Mindful Mommy

Your child likes the routine that you have set up and weaning can be scary and stressful for them. Make sure to keep an eye on toddlers who are slow to accept change. Avoid emotional battles over the breast. Slow-to-transition children need more time to accept change. Flexibility is important!

usually the most difficult to give up. Patience and consistency are key. Inconsistency will only delay the process.

Offer the breast less frequently and for shorter amounts of time. A delayed nursing session might even make a busy toddler forget. Don't refuse the breast, but don't offer it frequently.

Mix It Up

When it's time to eliminate that final nursing session of the day, rethink the bedtime routine. Give your baby a bath, read a story, give her a cup of water, brush her teeth, put on a lullaby tape, give a brief massage and kiss, and say goodnight. If you've weaned to the bottle, let Dad offer a bottle of water and initiate the bedtime routine.

Your partner can also spend time alone with your weaning baby. An afternoon out together, a walk around the block, or cuddling during storytime will distract a busy toddler from wanting the breast.

It's often helpful to eliminate the feeding cues that remind your baby that it's time to nurse. Sit on the couch instead of the chair. Face baby forward in the sling rather than toward your breast.

Mommy Knows Best

If you wean your child between six and nine months of age, you can begin to introduce a cup. Babies develop the ability to move objects from hand to hand in the middle of their bodies (midline) at around six months. By nine months, this skill is well mastered and babies are ready to manipulate cups with lids.

If your baby is six months of age, offer her a sippy cup with expressed breastmilk, 100 percent fruit juice, or water. A new taste, along with the novelty of the cup, will appeal to her. You can also replace a nursing session with the introduction of a new solid food. But remember to try new foods one at a time, and watch for signs of allergy.

Offer the cup following a feeding of solids and expect a mess. Remember: Babies are moist and they learn through their senses. Wet is good to a baby. Slidey, squishy, squirmy wet is even better.

Expect the cup to become a new toy for your baby. He'll throw it and expect you to pick it up (over and over and over). This game is not played to frustrate you, nor is it a sign of sippy cup palsy. Your baby is learning cause and effect ("If I throw it, you'll pick it up...every time!") and object permanence (out of sight is not out of mind). Both of these concepts are important for normal development, and you've just provided the right age-appropriate toy to teach them.

Age-Determined Weaning

Your weaning plan should take into account your child's age and developmental abilities. A child who is moving toward independence is more distractible than a child who has a much more predictable routine. Think about the ages and stages of your child when developing your weaning plan.

0 to 6 months: Wean from the breast to a bottle. Babies still have a need to suck. To avoid battles, offer the bottle to your baby when he is neither too tired nor too hungry. Babies at this age will often experience nipple confusion. Vary feeding positions, try different bottle nipples, and have someone else offer the bottle if he rejects it from you.

6 to 12 months: You can gradually replace breastfeeding sessions with solid foods and the introduction of the cup. Offer the cup more frequently. A pacifier can meet your baby's need to suck. Infants at this age are more distractible. A change in routines can help them transition from the breast more easily.

12 to 24 months: Your toddler is gaining independence and is mastering self-help skills. Toddlers at this age can now successfully manipulate a cup. Use the cup more frequently and begin to offer water in the bottle, if your child is using one. Your toddler is now eating table foods and has a varied diet. He sleeps through the night and doesn't rely on late-night feedings. This is the ideal age to introduce transitional objects for security (teddy bears and blankets) and to wean from the bottle. Teach your baby other ways to comfort himself.

24 to 36 months: Toddlers are active, curious, and on the go! You can substitute activities, like trips to the zoo or playground, in place of nursing. A change in routine will help eliminate nursing cues. Use a cup during cuddle times. Children love to listen to stories and make up their own. Replace nursing sessions with lap time in a different chair.

36 months and over: Children at this age nurse for emotional closeness. They prefer to play but still need to feel the safety of their parents. Invite your child's friends over to play more frequently. Have Dad offer days out with your preschooler as a change in routine.

If you have concerns with your baby's development with respect to his age, discuss your weaning options or plan with your pediatrician or lactation consultant. Again, you know your child best and are the most qualified judge of what methods will work for you and your family.

Transition from Breast to Bottle

Everything about gradual weaning should be gradual! Introduce bottles slowly and your little one should transition well. Bottle nipples aren't like human nipples, and infants suck differently from breast to bottle to cup. The nipple flow from a bottle releases milk more quickly, and depending on the nipple, in larger quantities. Look for signs of gulping and sputtering when your infant swallows. This indicates that the nipple flow is too fast. Switch to a

Mommy Knows Best

Watch out for ear infections! Bottle-fed babies are more prone to them. As you begin to wean from breast to bottle, feed formula or expressed milk mid-evening and water before bedtime. Milk that collects in the eustachian tubes is a perfect host for bacteria that will lead to painful ear infections.

slow-flow nipple or replace your current bottle nipple with a newborn size and flow rate.

Many babies experience nipple confusion when transitioning from breast to bottle. Often they'll refuse to take a bottle from their mother. Although the milk tastes and smells the same, the containers are different.

Transitioning off the breast is a perfect opportunity for Dad to begin feeding his baby. Ask him to offer milk or formula in a bottle or a cup. He can also offer solids if his baby is old enough to digest them.

Natural Connection, Natural Weaning

Some mothers decide to wait until their child gives them the cue. This is called natural weaning. It is a child-driven process that happens in baby steps usually between the ages of twelve months and three years. When you allow your toddler to set the rhythm, weaning happens naturally. Your hormone levels decline more slowly. There is little risk of baby blues or breast engorgement.

Mommy Knows Best

Did you know that some mothers can still express breast-milk long after they've weaned their babies or toddlers? In fact, some mothers still have small amounts of milk for up to two or more years following the weaning of their baby! It is not unusual and not cause for alarm.

A child's readiness to wean brings closure to the breastfeeding experience. When he initiates the process at his own pace, there are fewer power struggles. It allows him to have a greater sense of control and nurtures his self-esteem.

Mobile infants and toddlers are easily distracted by outside stimuli and will often wean themselves as they become more independent. While it's important to encourage your child's independence, it's equally important to meet his emotional needs. This is the "Don't offer, don't refuse" stage of weaning. If your toddler requests to nurse, you can allow it as often and for as long as you wish. But if you don't offer, your busy toddler will find other diversions.

Other Bonding Activities

Some babies have a hard time transitioning to bottles. So when you wean, make sure to pay a bit of extra attention to your little one. Babies still need to be close to their loving parents, both physically and emotionally. Let your baby know you're available to him in other ways besides breastfeeding. He needs the comfort of his mother's arms and plenty of time to cuddle.

Here are a few activities that will continue your nurturing relationship. (In fact, you may find that these activities are good for all nurturing relationships!)

- Color or draw together
- Cuddle
- Dance
- Do finger plays
- Go on a field trip
- Laugh at funny faces
- Listen to music
- Offer massage
- Read or tell stories to each other
- Recite nursery rhymes
- Rock in a chair
- Sing songs
- Tickle each other

Breastfeeding gave your child the most natural and healthy start to his or her life, but that was only the beginning. You'll spend the rest of your lives concerned with the health and welfare of your children as they continue to grow, learn, and become more independent every day. Through all the challenges that come with raising a family, have faith in yourself and your abilities, and remember, above all, to be loving and patient.

Appendix A

Additional Resources

THE FOLLOWING INFORMATION IS available to you so that you can further your understanding of the breast-feeding process. If you or your baby has specialized needs, speak with your OB, pediatrician, lactation consultant, or other healthcare professional. These professionals can offer you the best advice, based on your personal situation.

Breastfeeding Information and Support

American Academy of Pediatrics
P.O. Box 927
Elk Grove Village, IL 60007
(847) 228-5005
www.aap.org

International Lactation Consultants Association
1500 Sunday Drive, Suite 102
Raleigh, NC 27607
(919) 787-5181
users.erols.com/ilca/

La Leche League International
1400 N. Meacham Rd.
Schaumburg, IL 60168-4079
(847) 519-7730
www.lalecheleague.org

Lactation Education Resources
3621 Lido Place
Fairfax, VA 22031
(703) 691-2069
www.leron-line.com

Mothers of Twins Clubs
P.O. Box 438
Thompsons Station, TN 37179-0438
www.nomotc.org

Ted Greiner's Breastfeeding Web Site
www.geocities.com/HotSprings/Spa/3156/index.html

Web Sites

www.babycenter.com
www.babyzone.com
www.breastfeed.com
www.breastfeeding.com
www.breastfeedingresource.com
www.kidsource.com
www.naturalchild.com
www.nursingbaby.com

Breastfeeding Equipment and Supplies

Avent America
475 Supreme Dr.
Bensenville, IL 60106
(800) 542-8368
www.aventamerica.com

Hollister (Ameda-Egnell)
2000 Hollister Drive
Libertyville, IL 60048
(800) 323-4060
www.hollister.com

Medela, Inc.
P.O. Box 660
McHenry, IL 60051-0660
(800) 435-8316
www.medela.com

Books and Publications

The Art of Parenting Twins, Patricia Maxwell Malmstrom and Janet Poland, Ballantine Books, 1999.

The Breastfeeding Book, Martha Sears, R.N., and William Sears, M.D., Little, Brown and Company, 2000.

Breastfeeding, Pure and Simple, Gwen Gotsch, La Leche League International, 2000.

Caring for Your Premature Baby, Alan H. Klein, M.D., and Jill Alison Ganon, Harpercollins Publishers, 1999.

The Everything® Baby's First Year Book, Tekla S. Nee, Adams Media, 2002.

HHS Blueprint for Action on Breastfeeding, Department of Health and Human Services Office on Women's Health, United States, 2000.

The Nursing Mother's Companion, Kathleen Huggins, R.N., M.S., Harvard Common Press, 1999.

So That's What They're For!: The Definitive Breastfeeding Guide, 3rd Edition, Janet Tamaro, Adams Media, 2005.

Appendix B

Helpful Hints
for the First Year

Birth to 3 Months

- Sleep when the baby sleeps. These catnaps may be the only chance for sleep you get for some time.
- Use a car seat whenever you take your baby in a car.
- Your baby should sleep on his back to reduce the risks of sudden infant death syndrome (SIDS).
- Be sure not to let your baby get too warm. One light layer more than you would wear is plenty.
- Talk to your baby to stimulate brain development.
- Always support your baby's head when holding or carrying him.
- Never leave your baby on a couch or other high surface, as he could easily roll off.
- The human face is very interesting to your baby; give him lots of face time.
- Tummy time is a very important part of play. Your baby should spend some time on her belly every day to help build her neck muscles.

4 to 6 Months

- Be wary of toys that put weight on your baby's legs, as they may cause strain on undeveloped muscles.
- Do not start solid foods yet, as they may cause food allergies.
- Start babyproofing, if you haven't already. Mobility isn't too far off.
- You can't spoil your baby with attention. Remember to respond to her needs immediately so she will feel confident and comfortable when alone.
- Consider learning some simple sign language to teach your baby how to communicate before language abilities are developed.
- Make time every day to read to your baby, even if it's simply talking through a picture book.
- Have a car seat checkup. Your baby may have outgrown the car seat you've chosen.
- Juice is not recommended for babies. It simply leads to obesity and doesn't really offer any nutritional value to your baby's diet.

7 to 9 Months

- When starting solid foods, try one food at a time for several days to note any allergic reactions, such as rashes or irritability.
- Before moving your baby into a forward-facing car seat, check with your pediatrician to ensure that your baby is heavy and long enough for this to be safe.
- Check your home for low-hanging cords and unprotected electrical outlets. Your baby will be drawn to these at this age.
- Some sunscreens are safe for use on infants. Just be careful not to get any in your baby's eyes or mouth.
- Without going overboard, keep your baby's environment clean. Babies are very tempted to put things in their mouth at this age.
- Slings and backpacks are still great for getting around with your little one.
- Enjoy music with your baby. Different genres will inspire your little one to move and wiggle.
- Around this time, diaper changes may get a bit more hectic, as your baby won't want to be changed. Give your baby a special toy to play with to distract her during changes.

10 to 12 Months

- Zoos and petting farms are great treats for budding toddlers. Take your little one for a trip and tell her the names of all the animals. Just remember the importance of hand washing after touching animals.
- Babyproofing takes on a whole new meaning as your baby becomes more mobile. Take another look around your home for safety issues.
- Slings work well for carrying an older baby or toddler. They are also easier on your back than other carriers.
- Dry cereal is a mom's best friend during travel. Always carry a container of baby-friendly cereal with you in case hunger (or boredom) crops up.
- Don't be concerned if your almost-one-year-old is not yet walking. Many toddlers don't take their first steps until well after the first year.
- Play dates are great for older babies, but don't be discouraged if your baby doesn't want to play with a friend. At this age, you typically see parallel play, where the babies play next to each other with minimal interaction.
- Another car seat safety check is in order. Is your baby ready to turn around and be forward-facing? Do you know how to use your new car seat?
- Go through your medicine chest. Do you need to buy any new emergency meds to have on hand? Talk to your pediatrician about what medications you should keep at home.

Index

About the Authors

Suzanne Fredregill is a Certified Breastfeeding Educator, a Certified DONA Doula, a Certified Infant Massage Instructor, a Childbirth Educator, and a Licensed Master of Social Work. She lives in Des Moines, Iowa, with her husband Ray and their two children.

Kimberly Tweedy is a Certified Childbirth Educator, Certified Breastfeeding Educator, and a Perinatal Support Specialist. She holds a Bachelor of Science Degree in Nursing and a Bachelor of Arts degree in Sociology and Women's Studies. She has worked in the field of maternal-child health for the last 10 years. She lives in West Des Moines, Iowa, with her two children.

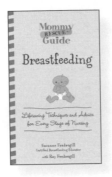
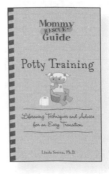
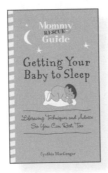
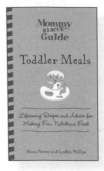